My Son, My Father, My Hero

My Son, My Father, My Hero

✦

One Family's Journey with Cancer

Larry and Delila Woodruff

iUniverse, Inc.
New York   Bloomington

My Son, My Father, My Hero
One Family's Journey with Cancer

iUniverse books may be ordered through booksellers or by contacting:

*iUniverse
1663 Liberty Drive
Bloomington, IN 47403
www.iuniverse.com
1-800-Authors (1-800-288-4677)*

*Because of the dynamic nature of the Internet, any Web addresses or
links contained in this book may have changed since publication and may
no longer be valid.*

*ISBN: 978-1-4401-9725-3 (sc)
ISBN: 978-1-4401-9726-0 (ebk)*

Printed in the United States of America

iUniverse rev. date: 1/30/2010

In loving memory of our son Larry Allen Woodruff.

Dedicated to Larry's four brothers:
Ronald
Donald
Rodney
Jason
For their support and love.

Dedicated to Larry's wife and two sons:
Kim
Blaine
Jeremy
For their unconditional love.

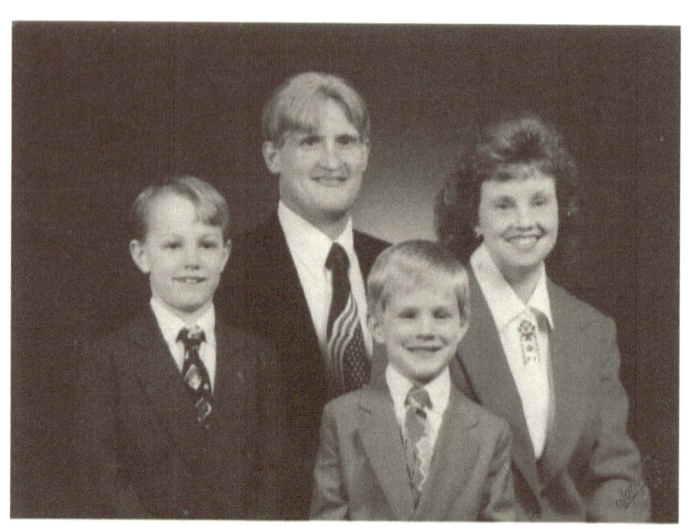

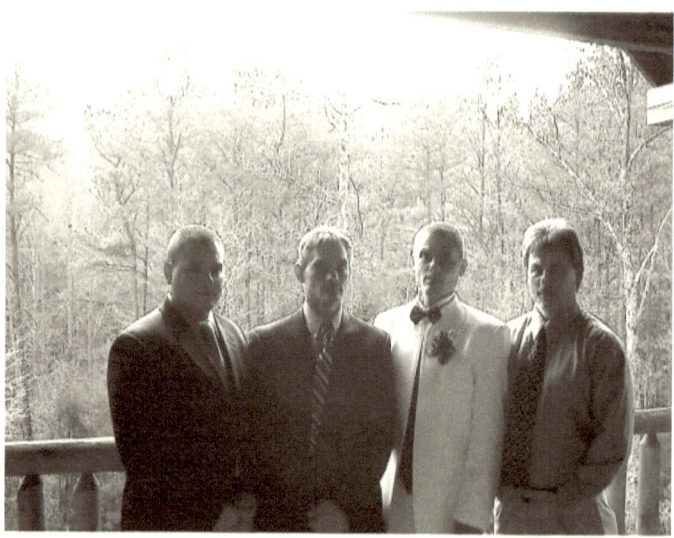

Contents

Preface

This is a story about the trials and tribulations of one family's long journey with the dreaded disease of cancer. The journey starts in 1984 and continues to 2004.

The story is told by Larry R. and Delila Woodruff, the parents of Larry A. Woodruff. Larry Allen has four brothers, Ronald, Donald, Rodney, and Jason. The book is based on the journal that was kept by his parents from the beginning of Larry A.'s illness. To ensure clarity in the book, we will refer to Larry R. as Larry Sr. to avoid confusing him with Larry A. Larry Allen and Larry A. are one and the same.

During our first week of dealing with this horrible nightmare, we met another mother whose son had cancer. She gave us some tips on how to get the best care and choices for our son. She told us to keep a daily journal of his medicines and treatments and record how he reacted to them. She also said that if a medical student tried to do a blood draw and couldn't get the blood after a couple of attempts, tell him or her to stop and get someone else to do the draw. When the doctors order a medical test, she told us to ask what they hoped to learn and what they would do differently after obtaining the results. And she told us to never forget that this was a teaching hospital and that the medical staff would do tests to learn different things concerning the illness.

The book is broken down into three parts. Part I starts in August 1984 and ends in September 1985, which is the beginning of the long journey. Part II picks up in September 1985 and goes to June 1987, which contains the major battle with cancer and includes entries from the journal we kept.

Part III starts in June 1987 and finishes in April 2004, when we deal with all the side effects of the radiation and chemotherapy.

This book was written to help other parents and families with loved ones who have had not only cancer but also other diseases that put a family in dreadful distress. The disease affects not only the patient but also everyone who is in direct contact with him or her. In our case, cancer affected Larry A.'s parents, brothers, wife, children, grandparents, aunts, uncles, cousins, and many friends.

On August 14, 1985, we faced the diagnoses of *cancer*, a word no family wants to hear. Larry A. fought the cancer as hard as any person could fight, but he also had help from a higher power. God and family were Larry's outside help, and with those sources he was able to defeat the cancer—only to find out ten years later that his brain was deteriorating from the very treatment that had saved him.

Larry Allen's normal weight before his illness was between 185 and 190 pounds. He had a healthy frame and stood six feet tall. He had blondish brown hair and was athletic, involved with track, football, wrestling, and gymnastics in high school.

In the following pages, see how Larry's family, with the help of God, fought his cancer, and see how they handled the brain injury from the cancer treatment and were challenged beyond all imagination.

Part I

Life is simply hard. That's all there is to it.
Thank goodness, the intensity of difficulty rises and falls.
Some seasons are far more bearable than others,
But none is without challenge.

Beth Moore

Chapter 1

✦

A Mother's Reactions

The room at Parkview Memorial Hospital became a room of morbid uncertainty, a room that would haunt me for the rest of my life. I wanted to cry—to scream at life for what it had done. Instead, I sat there showing no emotion as Dr. Frouts's words swam around in my head like unwanted parasites. His matter-of-fact attitude seemed cold. This wasn't the time to consider what made a man like him so detached, but I actually sat there and wondered. Perhaps my mind was searching for a way to cope with the news I had been given by pursuing senseless trains of thought. There was no doubt that I was in shock.

I will never forget that day: August 14, 1985. On that morning, the ringing telephone changed our lives forever. My son was in trouble. His voice on the other end of the line explained that he had fainted while taking a shower. From that very moment, our world as we knew it would never be the same. Life's traumatic situations can come at you in two ways: either one's world spins out of control, or one's world suddenly stops. Mine came to an abrupt halt, and suddenly the little things that made my world spin held no significance. What was I to fix for dinner? Should I go and buy that new purse? My car needed to be washed; the house needed to be cleaned.

I needed to stop by the grocery store and pick up a few things. What should I wear to work?

It just did not matter!

The sick feeling in the pit of my stomach told me that this was not happening to someone else; it was happening to me, to my family. Somehow, without preparing me at all, life had managed to deal me a card I did not want. This sickness was not in our family planning, and we had not considered it a possibility. Sure, I knew that humans all over the world faced difficult situations that were too traumatic to imagine. I suppose, like most people, I thought that really bad things happened only to others and that they would never, ever happen to my family, especially to one of my own children.

I sat there, dazed and confused, shaking on the inside but trying my best to remain poised on the outside. I couldn't fall apart, not in front of my son. If I lost it, he would sense that I saw his situation as hopeless.

Was it hopeless?

Larry Allen and I looked at each other disbelievingly. He had what Dr. Frouts called germ cell cancer. Here sat my son, facing the kind of news that only the aged should have to confront. He was too young for this—twenty-four, to be exact. He was the epitome of youth, vibrant and strong. *This could not be happening! The diagnosis…it has to be wrong!* Pastor Sims entered the room; I wondered how he knew we'd just received the worst news of our lives. He stayed and prayed with us as Dr. Frouts explained to Larry A. what was going to happen.

After Dr. Frouts left the room, a male nurse came in to do a blood gas analysis on Larry Allen. He asked me to hold Larry Allen's arm while he drew blood. The nurse told us it would be an uncomfortable procedure since the blood would have to be drawn from an artery instead of a vein. He went on to explain that this method provides a blood specimen for direct measurement of partial pressures of carbon dioxide and oxygen. It was also a way to quantify the patient's response to therapeutic intervention or diagnostic evaluation, which would monitor the severity and progression of a documented disease process.

I knew that this was only the beginning of the medical tests Larry Allen would have to endure. He would be prodded, probed, and cut…and God only knew what other things would need to be done. I knew this was a life-threatening situation for Larry Allen. I knew that our family would walk through this valley—the valley of death—together. I did not know the length or the depth of this valley, but I did know that we had just stepped over its threshold, where the dark unknown greeted us. What we would face was yet unknown. I was certain that the suffering and pain Larry Allen would have to endure would be, at times, unbearable for him. A mother never wants to see her child suffer. If I could have traded places with him I would have, but life does not give us that option. Instead, I would undergo my own suffering as I watched my child fight for his life without being able to do a thing about it.

The inner pain was crushing, and I had to escape, if for only a short time. I needed to call my husband, Larry Sr. He should know what was happening; and he would want to be with Larry Allen. I glanced over at the phone on the desk, not trusting myself to converse with my husband without going into hysterics. I made an excuse to leave the room. I found a pay phone in the lobby. My hands were shaking almost uncontrollably as I dialed my husband's work number. *God, if only I could awaken from this nightmare,* I thought as I waited for him to answer his phone.

Chapter 2

✦

A Father's Reactions

It was just another workday. I got up late and drove to work as fast as the speed limit allowed. When I arrived at North American Van Line (NAVL), a commercial and residential moving company that services the Midwest, the parking lot was packed with cars; the company was one of the largest businesses in Fort Wayne, Indiana. The building housed a thousand employees. I had been with NAVL for only six months. I was hired as a technical support programmer to help maintain the operating system on a large mainframe computer.

I had a few minutes to spare, so I went to the cafeteria and got a cup of hot black coffee and then made my way to the seven-by-fourteen-feet cubicle that I shared with a co-worker named Earl, a nice guy. We had plenty of space for two L-shaped desks and one bookcase. The morning work continued as usual. Occasionally, Earl and I would engage in small talk.

That afternoon, while I was editing a large file, the phone rang. I looked at the clock on my terminal; it was 1:58 PM.

"Larry Woodruff. Can I help you?" I answered.

It took only a few seconds for me to recognize my wife's crying voice. I felt myself go weak—I knew something was terribly wrong.

"It's Larry Allen," she sobbed before I could say anything. "His doctor says he's full of cancer."

She was crying so hard. I needed to be there—I had to get to the hospital. "I'll be right there," I told her. I hung up the phone without thinking or asking any questions.

I must have turned white. I could feel the blood draining from my face as I sat there in total shock. The news left me lightheaded and somewhat disoriented, but I managed to save all the updates to the file I was working on. The computer wasn't fast enough—the ten-second process seemed like a five-minute ordeal.

Earl was humming an upbeat tune as he shuffled through a small stack of papers on his desk, oblivious to my inner turmoil.

"I'm leaving," I told Earl as I walked out, not giving any explanations or waiting for him to respond. I didn't think I could say the word *cancer* without choking up.

My legs felt like rubber. I started down the long hall toward the parking lot. The hallway looked like it was four miles long. I was walking as fast as I could without running, but it was like slow motion. Getting to my car and driving to the hospital was like being in a bad dream.

I always parked in the same location, or close to it; otherwise, trying to find my 1985 Chevrolet Celebrity in a thousand-car parking lot would take some time. The twenty-five-minute drive to the hospital seemed like it took two hours. Every traffic light was red, and every car in front of me was moving slowly; but during the drive my mind raced with a hundred questions. *Who told you this? Are they sure it's cancer? Is it terminal cancer, or something that radiation treatment can take care of? Should we run more tests and get a second opinion?*

But the big question was *why*. Why did it have to happen to one of my sons? Why Larry Allen? He had it made now, with a bachelor's degree in computer science from Purdue University. He had a good job with a solid firm in Indianapolis, a new

Camaro, and a nice apartment close to his job. He was dating a really sweet gal, Susan. His future could not look any more promising. What more could a twenty-four-year-old need or even want? *How could this be happening?*

The taste of salt stirred my senses. I was crying and did not even realize it. The stream of tears had pooled in my mouth like a reservoir.

I pulled into Parkview Memorial's visitor parking lot and parked my car. The two-story brick edifice had, at other times, been a place of happiness for us. Parkview was where some of our boys had been born. Larry Allen had been the first.

Where does time go? I thought as I walked through the hospital doors and into the main lobby. *Who would have thought we'd be facing this in our lifetime?* It seemed like only yesterday that Delila and I got married and planned our future together. Our imagined future that was full of dreams and hopes; we expected to watch our children grow into young adults with dreams and hopes of their own. That was what we had dreamed; that is what we had hoped for; but that was yesterday.

Yesterday, I thought, as memories of those times flashed quickly through my mind.

Chapter 3

✦

Life Before

Told by Larry Sr., Larry Allen's father

I remember the sixties as the age of youth, as seventy million children from the post-war baby boom became teenagers and young adults. It was a time when the movement away from the conservative fifties resulted in revolutionary ways of thinking and the younger people wanted changes that affected education, values, lifestyles, laws, and entertainment. Elvis returned to the music scene from the U.S. Army, joining other white male vocalists like Bobby Darin, Jerry Lee Lewis, and Frankie Avalon. Motown Record Company distributed records specializing in black rhythm and blues and sponsored female vocalists and groups like Gladys Knight and the Pips, The Supremes, and Aretha Franklin. The Temptations became a big hit. Teens loved The Beach Boys and swooned over the new sensational rock group from England, The Beatles. Radio continued to be the primary way of listening to music, but the big development in radio was the change from primarily AM to FM. *American Bandstand* was soon to change that; now, teens could not only listen to their favorite songs but also learn how to dance to them.

New Haven, Indiana, was not much different from most other average-size towns in the early sixties. Roller rinks and the soda fountain were favorite hangouts for most teens. Bell's Roller Rink had an organ player who played some of our favorite tunes as we skated on shiny wood floors.

What really hit the town big was the new McDonald's restaurant on the west side of town. To signify its grandeur, large Ms that soon became known as the "golden arches" towered on each side of the building. The fifteen-cent hamburgers sold fast. When you placed your order, you could hear the beef patties sizzling on the grill and watch the frozen sliced potatoes turn into golden fries when they were dipped in hot grease. It was a haven for hearty appetites.

Gardner's Restaurant had carhops who took your order, and this was the place to cruise through. Another favorite eating spot was Briar Room, a restaurant where you could buy a fifty-nine-cent burger basket consisting of a hamburger and fries. On the weekend, a group of us would pile into a car and go to the drive-in for a buck a carload. Those were the days.

Eavey's Supermarket had a horn of plenty on its roof. You could see the wicker-horn, overflowing with fruits and vegetables, from a mile away—purple grapes, bananas, apples, pears, oranges, maybe even squash. It symbolized what most Americans worked for—the acquisition of plenty.

My father held a job at OIM Trucking Company and also served as a volunteer fireman. My parents bought a nice four-bedroom home. Along with my three brothers, Rex, Wes, and Lynn, I attended New Haven High School, and that's where I met Delila. Sonny and Cher's song "I Got You Babe" described us perfectly. After dating for two years, we were married at the New Haven Methodist Church. Delila's sister Carlyne and my brother Wes served as our attendants.

We didn't wait long to start a family. Larry Allen was born at Parkview Hospital in 1962; the twins, Ronald and Donald, were born in 1963 at the Lutheran Hospital; and Rod and Jason were born at Parkview Hospital in 1966 and 1973, respectively. We had always wanted a large, loving Christian family.

Larry was born with a bilateral cleft lip, and he underwent five surgeries before he was five years old. He also had reconstructive surgeries on his jaw in high school. Our family lived in New Haven and Fort Wayne, Indiana, until 1995; then we moved to Indianapolis.

Larry suffered two broken arms during grade school, one from practicing pole-vaulting in our backyard and the other from riding horses at his Uncle Al's farm.

Baseball was part of Larry's life; he played in Little League for seven years. I coached him for four years. Later, Larry became an umpire and umpired one of the games I was coaching. He also helped coach his youngest brother, Jason, when I had back surgery. He was a good-size boy, almost six feet tall and 175 pounds, with light brown hair and brown eyes.

In high school, he lettered in both wrestling and gymnastics. His math teacher said that he and Larry were learning together, because Larry was at the top of the class. He studied hard to make the dean's list in college. After college, he bought a new '84 Camaro, black with a "T" top; it was a beauty. He moved to Indy and went to work at the corporate office of Hook Drugs as a programmer/analyst.

Our fondest memories are centered on our home on Paulding Road, where we raised the boys. Delila was a stay-at-home mom. When Jason turned four, Delila taught gymnastics classes, and he attended the gym and swim program. The following year, Jason attended kindergarten.

Delila volunteered at Central Lutheran grade school, which our boys attended. She began teaching preschool part-time. At that time, I was working for NAVL, earning a decent income. We had our lives well laid out, like a clean load of laundry. But then life came along, rearranging the ideas we had so neatly folded, stacked, and stored away for future use. Walking into Larry Allen's hospital room was proof of that. I still couldn't believe this was happening to one of my sons.

There has to be a solution, a way to fight this, I thought as I stepped into my son's room. I could see that Larry Allen was having a lot of back pain. *Can't they give him something?* I wanted to wake up from this bad dream. I wanted someone to say that there had been a mistake and that we could all go home. We could spend the evening like we usually did. But I knew that wasn't going to happen. I took a deep breath and stepped over to Larry Allen's hospital bed. Delila was holding onto his arm as the nurse began preparing for blood work.

The phone rang—it was our son Rod. "Larry Allen hasn't made it home from the hospital. What's going on?" he asked Delila.

Delila looked over at me, heartsick. "Larry's not doing too well," she managed to say. "His test shows he has cancer." She hung up the phone. "He's on his way," she told us.

Moments later, Donald called, and I answered the phone. "This is Don," he said. "What's going on with Larry Allen?"

I couldn't bring myself to give him the news. I handed the phone to Delila and then stepped over to the window. Delila told him he needed to come up to the hospital, and then she explained Larry Allen's situation. A few minutes later, Ronald called from Indy, where he was sharing an apartment with Larry Allen. After Delila told him the news, he said he would be in Fort Wayne in the next few hours.

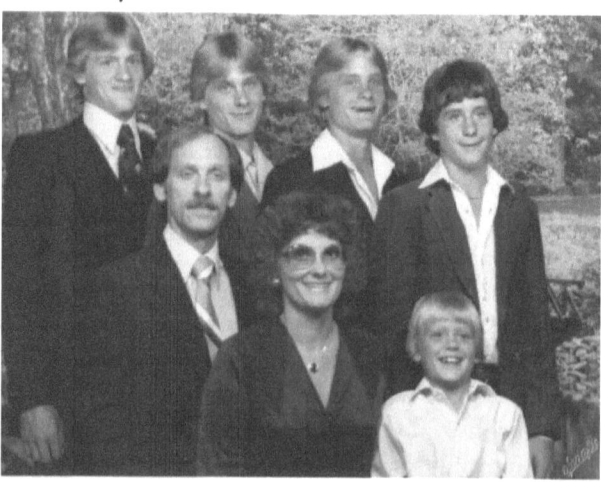

Chapter 4

✦

A Long Day

Told by Delila, Larry Allen's mother

It was one of the longest days of my life. Dr. Myers did not come in until around 9:00 PM. Larry's brothers and my mother were waiting with us. Finally, the doctor came into Larry Allen's room and introduced himself.

"It is advanced metastatic testicular cancer[1]," he told us, and then went on to explain: "I am sorry to say that it is in the advanced stages, and that Larry Allen is in real bad shape. The cure rate for this type of cancer is very good if it's caught in the early stages. His HCG[2] markers are 116,000, whereas the normal is 1 to 1.5. This is the highest I have ever seen."

It was news that I did not want to hear. I felt sick. I was hoping against hope that he could give us something to cling to—to fight for.

"There is a physician, a Dr. Einhorn, at the Indiana University Medical Center in Indianapolis who's had good

---

1 Advanced metastatic testicular cancer: small tumor on right testicle, two tumors on abdominal lymph nodes (left side, 5 x 10 cc; right side, 3 x 3 cc). Both lungs full of golf-ball-size tumors.

2 HCG (human chorionic gonadotropin) for gestational trophoblastic tumors and some germ cell cancers.

success in treating Larry's type of cancer," he said. "If Larry were my son, I would move him there for treatment."

"Then there is some amount of hope?" I asked, grasping at the small possibility that Larry Allen would make it through this.

"Who can say?" Dr. Myers responded. "I will give Dr. Einhorn a call tonight. You must understand, however, that if he feels Larry's case is hopeless, he may refuse to treat him. But I will see what I can do."

This 1 percent of good news didn't come to us until the next day. Larry Allen would be transported by ambulance to Indiana University Medical Center. Dr. Einhorn agreed to take Larry Allen's case.

After Dr. Myers left us, I put my hand on Larry Allen's arm. "We'll fight this," I told him.

He gave me a weak smile. "Sure, Mom," he said. "I guess I'm still finding all this hard to believe. When Dr. Frouts told me about the cancer," he said, shaking his head, "I'd been wondering what was causing my back problems. But I never would have guessed cancer."   Tears came to my eyes. "I know," I said, choking on the words and wishing for something to say that would give him a shred of encouragement.

"Why me?" he asked.

I fought back the deep emotion that was quickly surfacing, struggling to stay confident for Larry Allen's sake. But I wanted to go somewhere and sob uncontrollably.

Larry Sr. said, "We've all wondered that, son. Why?"

"I'm too young for this," he told us.

"We'll get through this together," his father managed to say. "Dr. Einhorn is supposed to be one of the best."

The room fell silent as we all tried to get over the shock of it all. Just talking about it was surreal.

A few hours passed, and I made arrangements with one of my close friends, Char, to keep our youngest son, Jason; she was Jason's godmother. Char didn't know what to say when I gave her the news. How would anyone know what to say in such a situation?

"Don't say anything to Jason about this," I instructed. "His father and I will give him the news later today."

By the end of the day, we had contacted family and friends, giving them the horrid news. Many came to the hospital to visit with Larry Allen. He was in a lot of pain, so we thought it best to allow only two at a time to visit with him. Everyone had cried so much by this time. Often, when I left Larry Allen's room, one of his nurses would give me a hug and cry with me. Nurses we didn't even know stopped us in the hall and said how sorry they were to hear about Larry Allen. I did not realize a person could hurt so badly and cry so much.

It was about 10:00 PM when I left the hospital. I had much to do to prepare for Larry Allen's transport to the I.U. Medical Center; I was going to be there with him. At home, we told Jason the news. He was very distraught, and I spent several hours comforting him. After he fell asleep, I packed my clothes for Indy and got Jason packed to stay with Char.

What would tomorrow hold? I wondered. I thought of Doris Days singing "Whatever will be will be." I shook my head. "No," I told myself. "I cannot be that indifferent to our situation: that whatever happens, we just sit back and let it happen. I won't take this with indifference. Survivors are fighters, and that's what this family will be: *fighters!*"

Chapter 5

✦

Off to Indy

Told by Delila, Larry Allen's mother

I cried when they put Larry Allen in the ambulance to transport him to the I.U. Medical Center in Indianapolis. He was given oxygen as well as a shot of Demerol to help manage the pain. There are comforts in familiarity, and leaving our home and Jason behind was overwhelming. I was unable to shake my deep despair and sadness. But the worst feeling was wondering if my son would return home with us.

My first impressions of the I.U. Medical Center were not positive. I felt we had made a terrible mistake in transferring Larry Allen. The center was much older and larger than Parkview Hospital. I doubted that the hospital was staffed well enough to give Larry Allen the one-on-one attention I wished for him to have. I wanted him to be treated with great care and consideration. I wanted him to be in a place where the medical staff did not consider him just part of their job, another task to complete before their day came to an end.

When Larry Allen arrived at the I.U. Medical Center, Dr. Einhorn and a group of doctors came in to evaluate his medical history and do a comprehensive examination.

During his first week at the I.U. Medical Center, Larry Allen had new medical problems due to the cancer treatment.

His white blood count was so low that the doctors worried he would start bleeding internally. The chemotherapy was affecting his veins, which made it difficult for the nursing staff to change his I.V. His hair was falling out from the chemotherapy. It was all over his bed and getting into his food. Rod cut his hair and then shaved the rest. I could tell that Rod was having a difficult time seeing his brother suffer like this. He tried to stay upbeat for Larry Allen, saying things to lighten the mood.

Our first conference was with Dr. Lerry; he did not give us much hope. "Larry Allen is in critical condition," he said. "He doesn't have long to live."

I looked over at my husband, whose look of anguish mirrored my own. I did not want to accept this news. I couldn't believe this was the end. "What are you saying?" I asked desperately. "Does he only have weeks, or months, or a year to live?"

Did I really want to know the answer?

"It's hard to say. Every cancer victim is different. He's in bad shape, and this type of cancer is very aggressive."

Larry Sr. asked, "Why have they not removed the testicle?"

Yes, why have they not? I thought. *That was where the cancer started.*

Dr. Lerry did not seem bothered by the question and answered, "The cancer needs to be treated first. As I said earlier, Larry Allen's condition is not good. We will remove the testicle at a later time. This type of cancer, in some cases, will trigger a brain tumor. We need to stop the cancer from spreading. There is one bit of good news that I can pass on to you. The latest lung X rays, to my amazement, did show some improvement."

The word *improvement* was all I needed to hear to reignite a spark of hope. The X rays before the first round of chemotherapy showed his lungs to be full of what looked like golf balls.

"You heard what the doctor said?" I asked Larry Sr. after we left the room. "His lungs have improved."

Larry Sr. remained thoughtful, his hands in his pockets, as he stood gazing out a window that overlooked one of the hospital's garden areas. After a moment, he turned to me. He looked so tired and worn. He was still recuperating from his own medical problems—he'd been admitted to the hospital a month earlier for multiple blood clots in his leg due to knee surgery.

"The chemo has been hard on him," Larry Sr. remarked quietly. "Maybe after it's all over and the cancer has been destroyed, his body will have a chance to heal, or at least recuperate. I really don't know what to think. They're not expecting him to live, you know. You did hear that—didn't you?"

Tears welled in my eyes. "Larry, I can't let him go—not without a fight." I walked over to him and laid my hand on his arm. "We've got to help him fight this. As hard as it may seem right now, I just can't throw my hands in the air and give up." Tears slid down my cheeks.

Larry Sr. turned from me and looked out the window again. "There are known medical miracles," he said. "Larry Allen's young, and who knows what his body will be able to withstand? Doctors have been amazed before, and this may be that one case that leaves them wondering."

"Larry Allen has a lot of support from friends and family. Sometimes that's what a person needs to get the determined will to live," I said. "I just want to make sure I do whatever it takes to help him."

Chapter 6

✦

Afraid

Told by Larry Sr., Larry Allen's father

The second week of September, they started Larry Allen on the second round of chemotherapy, which caused him to be very nauseated. For several days, he was able to eat without vomiting; but by the end of the week, he was vomiting a lot and sleeping most of the day. I couldn't help but notice how red and inflamed his left arm was from the I.V. Later, they applied moist heat and elevated his arm to help prevent any blood clotting. His blood pressure was very low. Delila's wish was to get Larry Allen home after his chemo treatments, but as I gazed down at his sleeping form, I wondered if that were possible, or even in his best interest. He'd lost a lot of weight, dropping from 186 pounds to 162. And I knew that by the time his treatments ended, he would have lost a lot more.

I began wondering just how thin a man could get and still survive. I honestly did not know. There were a lot of things about this cancer that I did not know, and feelings of helplessness consumed me. Delila mentioned buying books that would help us better relate to and understand what Larry Allen was facing. We would need to know what to expect in the days and weeks to come. Yet at times I wasn't sure I wanted to know. Larry Allen's future looked too grim. *How do you survive this kind of cancer?* I asked myself. Maybe God was listening, too.

As I sat there looking down at my son, wondering about it all, Delila came into the room with Rod. "They're going to let us take Larry Allen home as soon as they are able to get him off the I.V.," she said, removing her sweater and draping it over one of the chairs.

"How are we going to do that?" I asked, not sure I wanted him away from the medical attention he was receiving.

Delila quickly informed me, "The doctors and nurses are going to show us how to handle the I.V. line, check his blood pressure, and do anything else he may need. The rest of his treatments won't start up again for a while, and—"

"Wait a minute," I interrupted. "He needs medical attention, Delila. We can't possibly do all that he needs."

Larry Allen stirred. With difficulty, he managed to say, "I want to go home, Dad."

Delila added, "Visiting nurses will come out to the house and check on him. He wants to go home, Larry."

"I want him to be able to go home, too," I said, my voice strained with emotion. "But what if he needs immediate help? Then what would we do?"

I was afraid, afraid of so great a responsibility. I was no doctor. What did I even know about the medicines in my bathroom cabinet? I could barely even attend a child sick with a cold—let alone my son, who was struggling with terminal cancer.

Confused, I ran my hand through my hair. I wanted to take him home, but, at the same time, I wanted him to stay at the medical center.

"Larry?" Delila said, urging me to agree.

I looked down at Larry Allen. As if he could read my thoughts, he gave me a weak smile.

"You know I'm a chicken," I told him. "I hate needles."

Rod laughed. "Why do you think I'm here? The doctor and nurses are going to show Mom and me how to take care of the I.V. line."

Larry Allen was still smiling. Through it all, his disposition hadn't changed. He was the type of person who was always full of wit and loved to joke.

"Alright," I relented. "We'll get you home as soon as possible."

****

On September 14, Larry Allen was able to go home for the first time since starting his chemotherapy. It had been exactly one month and two days. It seemed like a year. So much had transpired, and the shock of it all still lingered heavily. But he was going home. The sun would rise another day for Larry Allen, and that would mean more to him than a million dollars. It would mean more to me than anything the world could ever give me. *Life,* I thought, *is such a precious commodity and so often taken for granted.* But like a lot of things, you don't often know its value until it is suddenly snatched from you. Life is precious, fragile, a gift, something to cherish. I would never look at it the same. Life was not to be wasted or lived without cause. From this day forward, I would do my best to make the most of my life. And from this day forward, I would cherish each and every day that Larry Allen was with us. How long that would be I did not know. But I did know this: I loved my son, and, according to what Paul wrote in I Corinthians, you have nothing without love. *A family's love*, I thought, *is truly what gives a man his life.*

PART II

EXCERPTS FROM OUR JOURNALS

Success is not measured by what a man accomplishes,
But by the opposition he has encountered,
And the courage with which he maintained
The struggle against overwhelming odds.

Charles A. Lindbergh

Chapter 7

◆

Home

Told by Delila, Larry Allen's mother

September 14, 1985

Home, we made it!

Larry Allen's weight is 149. He can't keep any food down and he has low blood pressure. He desperately wanted to be out of the hospital. For one month and two days, he has endured so many things.

I maneuvered the car into the driveway, handling it with ease. It was midnight. I'd driven from the hospital to our home on Paulding Road more cautiously than usual, trying to avoid the hard bumps in the road. Larry Allen sat on the passenger side of the car, and Rod had taken the backseat. Rod thought it would be easier for Larry Allen to get in and out of the car that way.

There was something about getting Larry Allen home that made me feel we were the winners of the first round. The fight had not left me, and I was still as determined as ever to see him get through this. No one could make me feel any differently. Not even the doctors, with their bleak and dismal prognosis, could make me give up.

I thought about my husband, Larry Sr., who, on the other hand, was still uneasy about his son being away from the doctors. If something went wrong and Larry Allen needed immediate help, what would we do? Larry Sr. would panic. *But if Larry could see his son's face now, all trepidation he had experienced would vanish,* I thought, watching Larry Allen's face light up as he glimpsed his home.

"Here we are," I said cheerfully as the car came to a stop. "You made it!" I leaned over and gave Larry Allen's shoulder a gentle squeeze.

"It's good to be home," Larry Allen said, gazing up at the two-story house he'd lived in for eleven years before moving out on his own.

Larry was feeling terrible. All of the treatments and chemotherapy he'd endured for the past month had made him extremely ill. It was impossible for him to keep food down, and his throat was sore from the constant vomiting. Would he ever feel like eating again? Even if he didn't want to eat, he would force himself to do so. If he were going to survive the next round of treatments, he would need to regain some of his strength.

Rod and I got out of the car and went around to the passenger side to help him into the house.

This was a big day, and our family had made all the necessary preparations for his care. Someone would be home with him 24/7. He knew we would try our best to see him through this. He'd been told that one out of every five people came down with cancer. In our family, the statistics held true—out of five siblings, he was the victim.

He was weak in the knees and felt wobbly. Two months ago, he wouldn't have imagined that walking would be laborious. But right now it took every ounce of his strength to get from the car to the house. The cancer had robbed him of all self-sufficiency. He'd just started out on his own—moving into an apartment, working his first full-time job after graduating from Purdue University—when suddenly, unexpectedly, the cancer came, stripping him of his independence. Will he ever know what it's like to be out on his own: to have a wife and children, or to buy his very own home? Larry Allen shared some thoughts with me about his girlfriend, Susan. What would become of their relationship? He wondered if he would even live another year. Would he see Christmas? It was only three months away.

Suddenly, feeling overwhelmed, he decided it would be best to take life a day at a time. And a day, he had discovered while in the hospital, could seem like an eternity.

As he stepped through the door and into the foyer, his father; two of his brothers, Donald and Jason; and his grandfather, Burness, eagerly greeted him. His grandmother, Helen, was not there; she'd died three months earlier from a massive heart attack.

His grandfather gave him a hug. Burness was still recovering from a laryngectomy (his voice box had been removed due to cancer of the larynx), so it wasn't always easy to understand what he was saying, but he managed to tell Larry Allen how good it was to have him back home. The hour was late, so they said goodnight.

Rod and I helped Larry Allen to bed. "I'll be right here if you need me," I told him. I hoped he would rest better at home. I gave him the necessary pain medication and then waited until he fell asleep before retiring in the recliner next to his bed.

September 16, 1985

The visiting nurse came to check on Larry Allen. His weight is dropping, and he has diarrhea. The nurse contacted the doctors and gave them a thorough report of Larry Allen's condition. Larry Allen does not want to check back into the hospital.

My heart was breaking. I was sitting in the chair next to Larry Allen's bed as the nurse telephoned the doctors. We'd been told that Larry Allen has the worst case of testicular cancer the medical center had ever treated.   "I'm   not going back to the hospital, Mom," Larry Allen whispered to me. "Not until it's time for my next treatment."

What was I to say? I didn't want him to be sent back to the hospital so soon either, but if it was life threatening, then he would need to go.

"I understand how you feel, Larry," I told him. "We'll do what we can to keep you here—you know that."

He said nothing more. The nurse hung up the phone and turned to us. "I'll be back tomorrow," she said. She gave Larry Allen a pat on the leg. "We'll see how things go for the next several days. We'll do all we can to keep you home."

"Thanks," Larry Allen said with a slight smile.

He looked exhausted, so I suggested he take a nap. "Jason will tire you out when he gets home from school. Best that you get some rest now. I'll fix one of your favorite meals for dinner."

"That'll be great, Mom."

I left the room before Larry Allen could see the tears streaming down my cheeks. *This shouldn't be happening to one so young,* I thought. *I need to be strong for him,* I told myself, wiping the tears away.

September 19–21, 1985

The visiting nurse came and said Larry Allen's heart rate was normal and that his lungs seemed to be doing okay. He took some bleomycin [3] from the oncology center at Parkview Hospital, and his hemoglobin[4] was 8.4. He is still vomiting a lot.

---

3   Bleomycin is an intravenous chemotherapy medication used to treat testicular cancer.

4   Hemoglobin is the protein molecule in red blood cells that carries oxygen from the lungs to the body's tissues and returns carbon dioxide from the tissues to the lungs. Normal in adult males: 14–18.

September 23–25, 1985

The visiting nurse found an irregular pulse, and Larry Allen's feet are slightly swollen. His weight has improved by two pounds, from 145 to 147.

September 26, 1985

Larry Allen was admitted to the I.U. Medical Center. An I.V. was started at 2:45 PM to hydrate him with fluid for twenty-four hours before any chemotherapy can be started. We arrived at the medical center at 11:15 AM, but the room was not ready until 4:00 PM. He was given the I.V. in the hall. The doctors could not feel the masses in Larry Allen's stomach when they examined him.

September 27, 1985

Larry Allen's blood markers (HCG) were 105, which was an improvement from the first two rounds of chemo. The third round of chemo was started at 11:30 AM. He vomited a lot that night. His weight was up to 154.

September 28–30, 1985

Larry Allen's weight has dropped to 150, and his blood count was 8.4.

October 2–3, 1985

Larry Allen continues to vomit. His hemoglobin is 11.1. Nurses turned down the I.V. to see if that might help. Doctors said that his kidneys are working and keeping up. They said they'd give him some Ativan to try and stop the vomiting; if that doesn't work, they'll run tubes down his nose. His throat is very sore.

October 4–5, 1985

This is the third day of chemo. Larry Allen had a hearing test that came out okay. He was very nauseated and vomited on the way back from Riley Hospital, which is connected to the Med Center by tunnel, after the test. He was also very dizzy.

He can eat a few ice chips. The I.V. was cut back a little more, and his urine output was off. We want to go home next week. He seems to feel a little better, but he has to stay in the hospital due to problems with his kidney. He can eat baby cereal without vomiting.

October 7, 1985

Larry Allen wants to go home for a few days. The doctor said he would release him if he could go all day without vomiting. Later, the doctor checked him over and discharged him at 9:15 PM. After the doctor left, Larry Allen started vomiting. He'd willed himself not to vomit so he could get out of the hospital and go home.

October 16, 1985

Larry Allen's weight is 135. He is glad to be home.

October 17, 1985

We're back at the medical center for another round of chemotherapy. An I.V. was started. A physical exam was done to compare with the exam of September 26; the doctor noted that there was a decrease in the multiple pulmonary metastases[5]. This was good news.

October 18, 1985

Round four of chemo, first day. Larry Allen's white blood count was low, and the doctors weren't sure about doing the chemo. Later they decided to go ahead with the treatment. Breathing test came back good.

---

5   Lung tumors that had spread.

October 19, 1985

Second day of chemo, and the results of the CAT scan showed marked improvement in the stomach and abdomen area. Larry A.'s hemoglobin is low, and he will need transfusions. I called Larry Sr. and told him about the transfusions. Larry Sr. will pick up the rest of the boys and get to the medical center as soon as possible. Ron and Don, who have the same blood type as Larry Allen, gave blood. Larry Sr. is also the same blood type, but he's been on blood thinners since he got blood clots after knee surgery in July. Larry Sr. is unable to donate, which upsets him.

October 20, 1985

Third day of chemo, and his pulse was up a little.

October 21, 1985

Fourth day of chemo. The doctors said there are still too many nodules in Larry Allen's lungs, so they can't operate. The stomach masses were smaller. Until they operate, the doctors can't be sure if the masses are cancerous or scar tissue. His testicle can still be shooting germ cells[6] into his body. He is vomiting green stuff. His blood count is low.

October 22, 1985

Fifth day of chemo. Larry Allen is still vomiting, and his weight is dropping.

"I want to go home," Larry Allen told me.

I blinked back the tears. "I don't know if they'll let you go home today. You'll probably need to stay on an I.V."

"I'll leave without the doctors' okay if I have to," he stated firmly.

I said nothing. I knew the doctors wanted him to stay on the I.V.; he was probably dehydrated from all the vomiting. The doctor also told me there was still a risk that the cancerous

---

6   Cells infected with cancer.

testicle would shoot off more germ cells before they would be able to surgically remove the testicle in six weeks. At the present time, Larry Allen's blood count is just too low to do the surgery.

"I want mashed potatoes and gravy," Larry Allen said, breaking the silence.

I smiled. Just hearing him say he wanted one of his favorite foods was a good thing.

Later that day, the doctors released him and told us if he dehydrated we should bring him back to the hospital. Larry Allen made it home; the gravy and potatoes were ready for him. The family happily watched him take every bite, but the joy soon dissipated when he couldn't keep any of it down.

Larry Sr. and I grieved tremendously to see our son go through the same ordeal time and time again. The next day, things had not improved.

October 24, 1985

We took Larry Allen to the Parkview emergency room. He was dehydrated, and his vomit had some blood in it. He was admitted, and the nurses immediately started the I.V. He was very weak and dizzy and mentioned that his legs ached. He was upset to be back in a hospital so soon.

October 25, 1985

Larry Allen's weight is 135, and he has a severe sore throat. He wants to handle as much of his illness as he can as an outpatient. He was discharged around 11:30 AM.

November 1985

Larry Allen has not been in the hospital for one month. This is the longest he's been home since he got his diagnosis of cancer. He sleeps a lot. His hair has started to grow out on the back of his head. He's excited about Christmas and wants to buy gifts for everyone.

He's worried about the big lymph node surgery in January.

December 3–26, 1985

Larry Allen was admitted to the I.U. Medical Center for testicle removal. His lung X ray showed improvement.

On the December 4, his right testicle was removed. The tumor was the size of a button. Dr. Donohue said it looked like the chemo had destroyed it. The surgery went well, and a CAT scan was ordered. The blood markers are 8.4—a miracle. The chemotherapy has worked on the cancer.

The CAT scan results showed that the stomach masses have shrunk. His lungs still have spots. The doctors will not make a decision about lung removal until they do surgery on January 2. Larry Allen's biggest fear is having his lung removed. But he seems to be handling everything else in stride.

His spirits have stayed positive, even when he is very sick.

January 2, 1986

We took Larry Allen to the Brown Derby Restaurant for lunch. He had tickets for the Pacers game today, but, due to pre-op for surgery, he will not be able to go. He insisted that his dad and brothers go to the game without him.

We checked Larry Allen into the hospital to get prepared for tomorrow's surgery.

After his pre-op, we were told that they might need to remove a kidney because of a tumor that is lying on a vein by the urethra tubes. This news was very upsetting. The positive news was that they would not remove the lung.

January 3, 1986

Surgery started at 8:00 AM. It took two hours just to prepare him. The entire family was there, and we were all scared of the outcome. Together, we went to the hospital chapel to pray.

We knew the surgery would be difficult, since chemo hardens the organs; the main artery would have to be peeled off the tumor. Nurse Gretchen promised to report to us about every two hours.

Surgery took eight hours, and then Larry Allen was taken to intensive care. The surgery was successful; both tumors were removed, along with the lymph nodes. We had not seen him now for ten hours, and worry had exhausted all of us. We were able to sit with him in the intensive care room. He'll now be fighting the risk of pneumonia setting in.

January 4–17, 1986

Larry Allen is in horrible pain and is taking pain medication. By January 6, he'd started running a fever. He can walk and sit up in chair. His brother Rod bathed him. The doctors told us that his internal organs are bruised, which is causing problems with urination. They are giving him shots of Valium, which is causing him to hallucinate. He is having bladder and body spasms.

On January 8, Larry A.'s tubes were unhooked, and the nose tube was removed. The pain shots were stopped. Yeah!

Dr. Donohue walked into Larry Allen's room, a smile on his face. "How are you feeling, Larry?"

Larry Allen smiled. "I made it through surgery. I won't complain."

"I have some good news," Dr. Donohue said eagerly. "From what I could tell in surgery, and from your progress, Larry, I think you're going to be one of the winners."

Larry Allen's face lit up, and tears of joy wet his eyes. I bit down on my bottom lip, praying that the doctor was right.

The doctor went on to say, "The blood markers were good. Your chart is showing that things inside are starting to work. I feel you're finally on the up side of this, and you'll start making progress."

Larry Allen's grin grew wider. He wasn't up to running in the halls and shouting the good news, so Rod and I did it for him. All the medical staff that was present gave us big smiles and said congratulations. Everyone involved with Larry Allen's case could not help but feel the joy of winning!

Ronald would come daily to the hospital after working all day and help with his care, while Larry Sr., Donald, and Jason would come and help on the weekends.

Rod reenrolled in college when Larry Allen's good reports came back.

Chapter 8

✦

More to Come

Told by Delila, Larry Allen's mother

February 7, 1986

Today is Larry Allen's birthday. We are so glad he's still alive and very proud of how hard he's fought to live. The family planned a surprise birthday party for tonight, inviting relatives, friends, and anyone who has helped out during his recovery.

Larry Allen felt really lousy today. He was vomiting and having bad headaches. I wanted to cancel the party but didn't have time to call everyone. It snowed really hard today; Rod shoveled out the driveway so people could pull in.

When everyone arrived for the party, Larry Allen was very surprised and tried hard to sit in a chair and be social. However, he had a terrible headache, and I felt so bad for him. Finally Susan, his girlfriend, got him to go upstairs to bed. Most of the guests stayed and partied, but I was not in the mood. I'm getting very concerned that something major is wrong.

February 8–9, 1986

Larry Allen is still feeling bad with headaches and vomiting and seems to be getting weaker each day. I think he's dehydrated again. Susan and Larry Allen left for Indy. She promised to keep a close eye on him. I looked over medical books to try and figure out what could be wrong with him, and I think it's a brain tumor. I decided not to say anything. I feel scared again.

On February 9, we went to Indy to drop off Grandpa Woodruff, my father-in-law, at the airport. He's flying to Florida to stay with his son and daughter-in-law, Wes and Peg. He'll be there for a few months.

Larry Allen almost passed out at the airport. He sat down for a while. Later, I told Larry Sr. that I thought Larry Allen had a brain tumor. He was shocked, and I explained to him what I had read on the subject. Larry Allen and his father are very close and have many things in common. Larry Sr. has suffered tremendously watching his son go through all this. He said he was angry with God and is no longer interested in going to church. I hated to hear this. I'm upset, too, but I need God to help us get through each day. I want to read the Bible and pray more, not less. I thought maybe God would keep him alive. I don't understand why all this is happening to our son. He has always been a son to be very proud of.

February 10, 1986

The rise of Larry Allen's blood markers should have been an indication that something was still terribly wrong. When Larry Allen saw Dr. Einhorn in an outpatient clinic, the doctor hadn't checked his results—if he had, it would have been caught. The markers were climbing 1,000 per day, and Larry Allen was having hearing problems, confusion, and trouble driving.

The pathology report was good from the lymph node surgery. Blood tests and chest X rays were done. The doctors thought that Larry Allen's headaches were stress-related. I didn't want to say I suspected a brain tumor in front of Larry Allen.

February 11, 1986

No phone calls from the medical center doctors. I started to hope the doctors were right, that the headaches were stress-related and would eventually stop happening.

February 12, 1986

Today is Larry Allen's great-grandmother's ninetieth birthday. We made plans to visit her at the nursing home. Larry Allen wanted to go, but he woke up with a really bad headache, and we thought it best that he stay home. My emotions were torn. I wanted to stay home with Larry Allen, but I knew I needed to go see Grandma. So I waited until Rod arrived home from college at 11:00 AM. My brother, Al, and I then left to go see Grandma Beth.

As soon as I arrived at the nursing home, I was paged. I had a phone call from Rod. He said that Dr. Einhorn had called and asked to talk to me. He then said that Larry Allen talked with Dr. Einhorn. Dr. Einhorn told him that the blood marker HCG was at 4,000 and that he needed Larry Allen to get to the medical center today.

The doctors suspected a brain tumor. They wanted Larry Allen to return to the I.U. Medical Center.

One of the hardest things I've ever had to do was go back into my grandmother's room and act like everything was okay. I didn't want to tell her the bad news on her birthday, nor did I want to upset her in any way.

I bent down and kissed my grandmother on the cheek. "I have to go," I told her. "Larry Allen's doctor telephoned, and they want him at the medical center right away."

Grandma Beth put a hand on my cheek. "It must be important. You go right along."

"I'll drive you," Al offered.

I tried to keep my composure. I walked out of the room, Al following quickly behind.

"Wait, Delila," he said as he caught up with me. "I can tell by the look on your face that something is terribly wrong."

For a moment I couldn't speak; the tight knot in my throat kept me from doing so. I took a deep breath and then told Al about the phone call from Larry Allen's doctor. "How can he survive this?"

I headed home, wondering how I would face Larry Allen and not fall apart in front of him.

Why is this happening after all he's already been through? He could have made it! But a brain tumor! Larry Allen is just not strong enough to go through another round of surgeries or chemo. He won't survive!

The entire ride home, I cried tears of anguish. It hurt deeply to see someone I loved go through such agony and physical torture. And then there was the darkness of death that seemed to want to snatch him from me.

When I got home, Jason met me at the door. "Rod won't let me go out and play," he said angrily, not knowing the reason why his brother was being such an ogre.

I touched his cheek. "Larry's sick again, Jason, and we have to get ready to leave and take him to the medical center. His doctor wants to see him right away. Do you understand?"

He thought for a moment. "Yeah, I know he's been real sick."

"Okay," I said gently, hugging him. "I need to make some phone calls."

Jason went outside to play with the dogs. I went to make the necessary phone calls. First I called our son Donald and asked him to come out and help take care of Larry Allen so I could do some packing. We called Ronald in Indianapolis; he would meet us at the medical center.

It breaks my heart to leave Jason again; he has been on a roller coaster for the past seven months, coming to Indy for the weekends with his dad, Donald, and Rod. I cannot leave Larry Allen at the hospital alone. He has such a love for God, and I feel my role is to help oversee his treatments and care for him.

After making the arrangements, I went upstairs. Larry Allen was stretched out on his bed. His six-foot frame looked frail; he'd almost wasted away to nothing during the months of treatments. I could say nothing; the pain was too great. I walked over to his bed and lay down next to him. I put my arms around him while he cried. I cried with him.

When Donald arrived, I left Larry Allen in his care while I packed and prepared to leave for the medical center. Larry Allen was vomiting and in a great deal of pain. Physically, my insides were in turmoil, and I was having a hard time focusing on all that needed to be done. Rod would take care of Jason, and Donald would take care of Grandpa Woodruff, which is a job of its own—he's taking radiation for throat cancer and must have transportation to and from the hospital in Fort Wayne.

Larry Sr., Larry Allen, and I left for the medical center around 6:00 PM. Susan and Ronald would meet us at the hospital. Larry Allen was in the backseat, shivering. "I'm freezing," he told us.

I covered him with our coats.

"I feel too sick to make any medical decisions," he told us, his voice weak and barely audible. "I trust you and Dad's judgment, but please promise me you won't keep me alive on machines."

I cringed at the thought of needing to make such a decision. Larry Sr. clutched the steering wheel until his knuckles turned white, his insides knotting up. We both promised him that we would do as he requested.

Ronald and Susan met us in the emergency room. The nurse immediately hooked Larry Allen up to an I.V. After the medical staff checked him over, they said he was severely dehydrated and possibly going into shock.

Was this the end?

Ronald would come up after work, and if Larry Allen was not doing well, we would spend the night at the hospital.

February 13, 1986

A CAT scan of Larry Allen's head was done around 7:10 AM to verify that it was a brain tumor. Dr. Nick is the doctor of oncology this month. Dr. Donohue was out of town, so we had no choice but to use Dr. Nick. I did not care for him. Later that morning, they came to take Larry Allen for radiation treatment. I refused to let them do this until the doctor explained the CAT scan results.

Dr. Nick reported a brain tumor on the left side. He suggested radiation and a different mixture of chemotherapy. I agreed to one round of chemo so I could see how Larry Allen handled it. I didn't feel he could go through another round of chemo—not if he got really sick on the first round.

The radiologist showed us the tumor on the CAT scan; it was the size of a tennis ball. Swelling in his brain was causing the vomiting and migraines. The brain tumor can activate cancer through his body. He will need five weeks of radiation and chemo as a preventative. The radiologist was shocked that Larry Allen had not had a seizure due to all the swelling in the brain but did feel there was a good cure rate using radiation treatment.

First day of chemo and radiation

Larry Allen was told that his hair would grow back. They did the markings on his head and gave him the first treatment. He was exhausted, and his head was hurting. He was also given steroids to help treat the brain swelling. He had excessive vomiting and dry heaves.

February 14, 1986
Second day of chemo and radiation

Larry Allen vomited a lot and had a racing pulse. They increased the pain medicine. We rub his back a lot to help relieve the back pain. He has not eaten since Tuesday and has headaches.

February 15, 1986
Third day of chemo and radiation

Larry Allen is experiencing confusion and cannot remember what we are saying. He says he can't concentrate. His headaches are the same. He is getting weaker, and his legs and back hurt.

February 16, 1986
Fourth day of chemo and radiation

A depression of the bone marrow was done today. Larry Allen is to avoid anyone with cold and flu symptoms. Dr. Nick met with Larry Sr. and me; he said Larry Allen was not responding to treatments as well as had been expected. He explained that radiation causes the brain to swell, and they will need to increase the steroids.

His stomach pain, and the pain on his right side, is getting worse. More X rays were taken, and no blockage showed up, but he is having trouble voiding (urinating).

February 17, 1986
Fifth day of chemo and radiation

Larry Allen is vomiting a lot and cannot keep down any pills. He has been very weak and fell asleep on the radiation table. He fainted in the bathroom, bumping his head and bruising his knees. Usually, he tells us when he is feeling dizzy and we are able to give him support, but this time there was no warning.

They are giving him Demerol for nausea and headaches. The nurse told us there are approximately twenty chemo patients on the same floor.

Larry Sr. told me he has not given up but realizes that Larry Allen could die this time. Larry Allen wants to know if he is treating all of us okay. *Dear father in heaven, it's breaking my heart to watch him suffer so much, and he wants to know if he's treating us okay?*

I asked Dr. Nick to call in a neurologist. I suspect the cancer has metastasized to the spine, and there will be no other treatment to save him. Dr. Nick refused to call another doctor onto the case. He also refuses to recognize Larry Allen's malnutrition and start a feeding tube. I'm getting very upset about the way the case is being handled. He is deteriorating so fast.

February 20, 1986

The radiation machine was malfunctioning today. They did not want Larry Allen to miss any treatments, so they used the cobalt machine. I feel uneasy about this. When I asked if the cobalt treatments would permanently damage the head for hair growth, I was told that they would not.

The pain is bad in his side, and he is vomiting a lot. The I.V. in his hand is swollen due to infiltration, and I worry about a blood clot forming there. We have been using moist heat on it.

Dr. Nick still refuses to administer a feeding tube. I'm getting very discouraged and frustrated. Larry Allen is getting worse every day, and I don't know what I can do to turn all of this around. I wish I knew more about everything.

Dr. Donohue came in to see Larry Allen and agreed that he has a severe nutritional problem that could destroy him. I told him what I told Dr. Nick about a feeding tube. Dr. Donohue suggested that I tell Dr. Nick that I want him in on the case. I feel hopeful that Dr. Donohue will straighten out the situation.

Thank you, Jesus, for Dr. Donohue's concern. Dr. Donohue is back on Larry Allen's case. Otherwise, I'm sure Larry Allen would not last much longer.

Dr. Donohue and I talked at length about when the brain tumor had started. We both felt it had started around August 1985. At that point, Larry Allen had complained of eye problems, and Dr. Einhorn had mentioned the possibility of a brain tumor. When they ran a CAT scan without contrast materials, due to his kidney damage, no tumor showed. Dr. Donohue concluded that the tumor started growing sometime after the chemotherapy ended.

Ronald works during the day and spends the nights with me at the hospital. Larry Sr., Donald, Rod, and Jason come on Fridays for the weekend and help care for Larry Allen. Conn, Larry Allen's friend from grade school and college, comes and visits him as well. This is when Ron and I sometimes take a break to go back to his apartment and get cleaned up.

Weekends, I spend time with Jason at our apartment in Indy. Larry Sr., Donald, and Rod take turns at the hospital. If Larry Allen is not doing very well, however, we all stay at the hospital.

The reoccurrence is hard on all of us for different reasons. It's discouraging for Larry Allen; he went through so much chemo and so many surgeries and is still fighting for his life. It's heartbreaking for Larry Sr. to know that one of his sons is experiencing more pain than any person should have to go through; and he can't bear the thought of losing him. Ronald is exhausted from working days and being at the hospital at night. Donald is still responsible for Grandpa Woodruff's needs. Rod feels torn, since he started college after he thought Larry Allen was cancer-free. Jason knows his family will be separated in two different towns for many more months. I'm concerned about Larry Allen's pain and what treatments will be added to his hospital stay. I'm worried about the family back home in New Haven. Each day at 3:30 PM I think about Jason coming home from Central Lutheran School and how much I miss not being there.

Chapter 9

✦

Complications

Told by Delila, Larry Allen's mother

February 21, 1986

The radiation equipment is still not working, so cobalt treatments were given again today. A spinal tap was done to check for bacteria and cancer. All the steroids could be masking a fever. His pain could be bladder backup, since he is having problems voiding. Kidney stones are another possibility, and the kidney doctor said Larry Allen has poison in his body.

We are not happy with Dr. Nick. We feel he gives dumb guesses when we ask questions. I have demanded that Dr. Donohue stay on his case, and I want Dr. Nick removed completely. He agreed to call Dr. Donohue, but Larry Allen's chart shows that he called only a renal doctor. One of the nurses said something must be done about nutrition. Dr. Nick refused to do the food line[7] because of Larry Allen's low blood counts. The counts won't matter if he starves to death! I'm getting angry at the system. This is my son lying here, getting worse each

---

7   A food line or feeding tube is a medical device used to provide nutrition to patients who cannot obtain nutrition by swallowing.

day. *Larry Allen tries so hard to be so damn brave*, I said to myself.

Later, Dr. Donohue gave Larry Allen a 50 percent cure rate. This was encouraging, and Larry Allen felt less tense knowing that Dr. Donohue is in charge of his case.

There was blood in his vomit today, and the pain in his side was worse. He worries about what his dad and brothers are thinking. The renal doctor reported that the ultrasound shows urine backup. The chemo nurses tell me they think this is due to steroids. Dr. Donohue suspects nerve damage. Larry Allen's back is starting to swell. He is so weak that Ronald had to help hold and support him when they did X rays and other tests. Larry Allen always gets worse on Sunday nights after his dad and brothers return to New Haven.

February 22, 1986

A neurologist came to see Larry Allen today. He did not understand his case due to the lack of information given by Dr. Nick. Ultrasound results showed an enlarged kidney. The myelogram came back okay.

Dr. Nick said we could use a pain block on Larry Allen after determining the cause of pain. The doctors inserted a catheter to drain his kidneys.

February 23, 1986

Larry Allen's abdomen is very swollen, and no one seems to know what is causing the swelling. Morphine pills were given for his pain.

February 24, 1986

Radiation was cancelled today due to Larry Allen's poor condition. He was given two units of blood. I'm very upset that I wasn't told a few days ago about the blood he'd need. Dr. Nick knows we don't use random blood—only blood from our donors. Larry Allen moans a lot in his sleep. He has shakes and chills, and he is weak and runs a temperature of 101.1. His abdomen is continuing to swell, and the side pain is worsening. I refuse to okay a pain block until they determine the cause of the pain, so they increased his pain medication. His kidney and bladder are doing okay today, but he is having a lot of pain in his back and neck. They said he could be bleeding internally.

February 25, 1986

Larry Allen's feet are swollen, and he can't relax or sleep. He acts hyperactive, and they feel this is due to all the medications; they plan to cut back. We were told to arrange for blood donors. The radiologist said that if his blood count doesn't come up, they'd need to delay radiation. Dr. Donohue says I should always keep in mind that the top priority is to kill the cancer. When a patient has as many complications as Larry Allen does, it's important to keep treating the cancer if possible. I was glad to hear that; he is developing so many complications, and it's so confusing.

February 26, 1986

Dr. Donohue says that Larry Allen has ascites and staph infection. Ascites is the abnormal accumulation of fluid in the spaces between tissues and organs in the abdominal cavity. He is spitting up blood and having a lot of fluid retention. The swelling in his stomach is moving higher. He is unable to sleep and has no bladder control. He is very upset about wetting the bed and nearly broke down and cried. He said he was so embarrassed about it. I told him it was due to all of the drugs. Dr. Nick reported that Larry Allen is in very poor condition and at great risk for three to four days because of his blood counts. He could start bleeding at any time. I feel that Larry Sr. and I should both be at the hospital around the clock. They can't draw the fluid from his stomach due to a high risk of infection. The doctors agree that if they drain the ascites, it will refill more than before. I was told that the ascites was caused from the lymph node dissection and the lack of nutrition in his blood.

February 27, 1986

Today's radiation was canceled due to Larry Allen's low blood counts. They're going to start a morphine I.V. to control his pain, which is so bad he can hardly breathe. I feel like the fluid is smashing his insides. Some nights, I feel he won't make it through until morning. It is horrible. I don't want to lose him, so I refuse to give up.

February 28, 1986

He started having nosebleeds. Radiation was canceled again because his blood counts are not going up. One unit of blood was given. His stomach measures thirty-seven inches.

March 1, 1986

This was a bad day. Larry Allen was running a temperature and had terrible diarrhea—he went all over the bed. He gets a slight headache if he sits up for very long.

March 2, 1986

Today, our family and Dr. Einhorn decided that Larry Allen wouldn't have any more chemotherapy. Dr. Einhorn feels Larry Allen's body is too weak, and he's afraid Larry Allen is headed for leukemia since so much of his bone marrow has been zapped. He also feels that Larry Allen still has a good chance of beating the cancer. The doctors want him to try eating more. We keep telling them that there is no room for food in his stomach because of the ascites. I feel no one is listening to us; they don't seem to comprehend this.

Larry Allen's stomach size increased today to 37.5 inches. His bed was elevated to help him breathe.

March 3, 1986

Radiation was canceled again due to low blood counts. The fluid in his stomach is moving higher. He is very uncomfortable and can't lie flat. Almost all of his hair has fallen out. His feet are badly swollen, and blood spots are appearing on his skin. His stomach has been so swollen that he has stretch marks. His blood platelets are down again. An X ray showed that his lungs are being pushed up from the fluid. If he has pneumonia, as they suspect, it will not show due to the fluid inside his body. They won't drain all of the fluid from his stomach because they feel it will cause his stomach to refill faster. A culture of the fluid will be tested again.

His platelets must be fifty thousand due to radiation treatments. I pray that someone figures out what to do and gives him some relief. It is a nightmare watching him suffer this way. We don't leave the hospital anymore unless a family member is with him.

March 4, 1986

Larry Allen was put on a special diet that may help control the fluid. His feet are still badly swollen. His urine output is too low, and the doctors are concerned that his kidneys are shutting down.

He is very depressed and in a lot of pain. He doesn't want to eat or drink because of the pain it causes afterward. We have so many doctors on the case, and each one is guessing something different. Since Larry Allen has taken a turn for the worse, some of the doctors avoid me. I let them know this is not acceptable—I expect to be kept informed.

March 5, 1986

Blood markers show 132.7, so the treatment for the cancer is working. Radiation was given, but with low counts. Larry Allen's feet are still swollen badly and very uncomfortable.

March 6, 1986

Larry Allen's stomach measures thirty-nine inches, and he is having a bad case of indigestion. He walked a little and sat in the lounge. His stomach culture came back okay.

March 7, 1986

Radiation was given today, but Larry Allen's counts are still very low. I put wet, warm cloths on Larry Allen's forehead. After packed blood cells were given, he began to have chills. This could be a reaction to the pack cells; he has had so many recently. Plus, the bedsores on the end of his tailbone are bad. He is running a temperature and is still very depressed. They removed some of the fluid from his stomach, but it refills. No one knows what the fluid is.

March 8–13, 1986

Today—finally—a feeding tube was started through Larry Allen's nose. A nurse told me that someone in the family should be at the hospital at all times due to Larry Allen's condition. We have already been doing that as much as possible. He was given a blood transfusion. A chest X ray shows more fluid than the last time. When fluid is removed, his stomach refills with the same stuff. He experiences vomiting and diarrhea every time they give him Hyperale[8] in the food line, so they stopped the Hyperale. He took another turn for the worse and could hardly get his breath. He was having a lot of back pain. His stomach has gotten larger. The catheter did not get much urine out. His morphine dose was increased. The I.V. site was changed to the other side of his chest. Larry Allen is incoherent at times. Any type of surgery would be very risky due to his high potassium levels, which could cause cardiac arrest. Radiation was given. I called and talked to Larry Sr.

---

8   Hyperale is a liquid nutrition that is fed through a food line in the stomach.

off and on through the night. I was so afraid that Larry Allen would not make it through the night.

The next day, Larry Allen received radiation treatment. His face is discolored, like a dirty tan. His breathing is worse due to fluid backup. His kidneys have shut down. He is spitting up blood and running a temperature. A medical student informed us that all the doctors are talking about Larry Allen's case, and they are not sure what to do. They feel the fluid may be caused by an untied lymph node from a previous surgery. A shunt may cause all the fluid to run out when they open him up. Larry Allen is asking what the doctors are planning to do for him next. I won't tell him they don't know what to do, or that some of the doctors have given up on him. He has fought so hard to live; any discouraging news, especially from his doctors, would be too hard on him.

March 18–25, 1986

Dialysis started today. Larry Allen was given four days to live if the poisons in his body were not flushed out. Treatment took three and a half hours. He vomited during the treatment. The dialysis technician was good with him and observed him closely the whole time.

Fluid in his lungs was suctioned out. Larry Allen wants the respirator turned off and the nose tubes removed. They took him around 9:00 AM for more tests. Larry Allen does not want any more tests—he's sick of them—but I talked him into one more. They let Ronald go with him to help keep him calm. The doctors suspect renal blockage. The test showed holes in the urethra tubes that were caused by the massive amounts of steroids given to Larry Allen.

Larry Allen has a terrible time having any tests done. He is so thin, and lying on the testing table makes his pain worse. I now require a good reason for the tests they want to do. Larry Allen is also refusing to have so many tests done. Dr. Donohue respects his wishes.

The doctors need to do surgery to repair his urethra tubes, which have ruptured and are allowing urine to get into his body. Surgery went well, tubes were put in, and his kidneys are draining well. Larry Allen is now able to breathe without the respirator. His liver counts are coming up slowly. His heart rate bounces up and down from 50 to 110. The side effects of the fungus drug are chills, shakes, sweats, and fever and kidney damage.

His weight is 132 pounds. He has blood in his stool and is short of breath. He does not want to be put back on a respirator, even though the doctors explained that it makes it easier for him to breathe. We had to explain that we promised Larry Allen at the start that we would not go against his wishes.

On March 24, at 1:00 AM, he had to have an oxygen mask put on. The lower part of his lung was not working properly. Due to brain swelling, he was give hydrocortisone. Larry Allen can't sleep. Dr. Leaper feels it is because breathing on his own is too difficult.

He is having chills and is disoriented. He may have pneumonia. All the doctors are saying that it is the worst case of malnourishment they have ever encountered.

He is in the intensive care unit, and I was surprised at how many machines were brought into the room. Larry Allen is having a difficult time. His breathing and heart rate are not good. He is grouchy and won't stay covered up. This is not like him; he is always very modest. A shunt is pumping fluid out. He won't eat and says he doesn't care anymore if he gets well. I asked him about going home, and he said no. I feel his spirit has been broken. He was always determined to get out of the hospital as quickly as possible.

I feel like part of me is dying each day as I watch Larry Allen suffer and dwindle away. God help us.

March 27, 1986

His feet are swollen, and his stomach is still thirty-five inches. He had a milk shake and tried to read the sports section so he'd be able to talk with his brother Rod when he came to visit.

Larry Allen has been in intensive care for a month, and they feel he has I.C.U. psychosis. He is not giving off enough carbon dioxide, which causes disorientation.

Ronald and I went home late to change clothes and stretch out for a few hours. I lay down, but the phone immediately rang. A nurse explained that Larry Allen had pulled the overhead light out of the wall and was crying and very upset. He hadn't harmed himself, but when we arrived he said he went nuts and feels like he is floating. He keeps asking why he is here.

April 2, 1986

I put a sign above Larry A.'s bed that said *Caution: Crisis in Progress*. I requested that the medical doctors and students address Larry A. by his name. He is not a number on a chart. He is person and needs to be treated with respect.

They have replaced temporary stents with more permanent ones. Dr. Mooch listed ten major health problems that Larry Allen is dealing with:

1. Brain tumor
2. Ascites—fungus
3. Pneumonia—fluid on the lungs
4. Kidney damage—quantity and quality of urine
5. Urethra tubes—kidney and bladder tubes
6. Nutrition
7. Liver function
8. Diaphragm—damaged form the ascites
9. State of confusion
10. Diarrhea

Easter 1986

Today Larry Allen wanted to go outside in a wheelchair. He hasn't walked since being admitted to intensive care. The nurses said they'd never taken an I.C.U. patient outside, but if the doctors gave them the okay, they'd help us. He was so excited, and all of us were with him. Once we got the doctors' okay, we put him in a wheelchair and went to the front of the hospital to see the view. We were out only for a short time. He had a very bad case of diarrhea, and when we looked down, we saw that it had gone everywhere. The boys got a bunch of paper towels to clean the cement, and we took Larry Allen back inside and cleaned him up.

Spring Break 1986

Jason was going to spend the week with me. Ronald was going to try to get a few days off to play with Jason. Ronald and Jason had bought remote control cars a few weeks earlier. My sister Carlyne came on Monday and spent the night with Larry Allen. I was going to the apartment for a while so Jason and I could get cleaned up. We stayed at the apartment for a few hours and slept. I had a bad migraine.

The next day, Larry A. was going to have more tests done. Carlyne arranged to stay with him, while Jason and I went to lunch. During lunch, I felt uneasy; I wanted to get back to the hospital. Call it mother's intuition, but after eating I headed back to the hospital to check on Larry Allen. I called the apartment to see if Ronald was off early to do something with Jason. However, Ronald was home—he'd had a grand mal seizure at work. An ambulance took him to another hospital in Indy. The doctors there wanted to admit him and run some tests. Ronald refused to stay and would not let anyone call me due to Larry Allen's deteriorating condition. Ronald felt the family couldn't take much more. He did say, however, that he felt exhausted from the seizure.

Ronald didn't want to be an added burden since Larry Allen's condition was so dire, but I was worried about Ronald's seizure and didn't want to ignore it. After I talked with Dr. Donohue, we made arrangements for Ronald to see a neurologist at the medical center. In the meantime, I was to take him to the emergency room for testing, and they insisted that Ronald be admitted for a spinal test. Dr. Donohue also informed us that Ronald had a high chance of experiencing another seizure in the next forty-eight hours.

Jason was too young to get into the I.C.U. to see Larry, so he played with his remote-control car in Ronald's room. I felt so bad that Jason had to spend his spring break at the hospital, but there was no choice. I missed Jason so much when he wasn't in Indy.

Ronald was admitted on the same floor as Larry Allen, but Larry was in the I.C.U. Ron didn't want to be treated as a patient, so he came to Larry Allen's room and sat with me. All that was on my mind was Ronald. Would we see another son suffer? I borrowed reading materials so I could learn everything I could on all types of seizures and their causes.

Additional Thoughts

Dave, a medical student who had been on Larry Allen's case since the first month, had become very important to us. Dave could get an I.V. and needles into Larry Allen's veins on the first try. This was no easy feat since Larry Allen's veins had become very hard from the chemotherapy treatments. I called Dave "Larry's guardian angel." If another medical student tried to get a needle in and couldn't get it after the first few tries, I would tell them to stop, and I would try to find Dave. Sally, whose son was also being treated for cancer, told me to draw boundaries. Students will keep trying over and over again—they like the experience.

The Cancer Research Center (C.R.C.) was the special wing where Larry Allen stayed after his first few weeks at the medical center. It was a small wing, with about nine private rooms for patients and family members. This became our home, and we knew all the nurses on the floor. One nurse, Judy, was our favorite. She was like a mother to us all. She taught me how to read Larry Allen's test results.

Rod and I studied Larry Allen's chart each night. I also had copies made in case we needed them in Fort Wayne. Every Friday night, Judy would have things for Jason to do.

Susan came almost daily to visit and help care for Larry Allen. Many family members and friends would help during the week and at night. One of our nephews, Brad, came at night during the week. If Larry Allen were not doing well, he would stay by his bed most of the night until it was time to leave for work the next morning. Brad and his wife, Koreen, stayed many weekends to help out.

Conn and Connie were very supportive. Conn would sit with Larry Allen so we could leave the hospital to eat and clean up. He would also watch a ball game with Larry Allen. Connie made a lot of dinners for us. She also donated blood. Grandma Linker called frequently during his bad times or surgery. She also stayed for a few days at a time to help and keep me company.

Grandpa Woodruff was trying hard not to be a problem for anyone. Grandpa helped Ronald and Larry Allen with the financing of their apartment in Indy.

Al and Carol were really great to all of us. Al ran Rod to the medical center in the middle of the week if Larry Allen took a turn for the worse. Carol called daily to help with some of the decisions and was very supportive. Al and Carol also came on weekends to help out.

Larry Allen felt more secure with family and friends at the hospital, so we made certain that a family member was with him at all times.

Emmanuel Lutheran Church brought many meals to the house for Larry Sr. and the boys.

We could not have faced these trying times on our own. Thank you for your prayers, your support, and your very kind deeds. May God bless all of you!

Chapter 10

✦

Last Radiation

Told by Delila, Larry Allen's mother

A day before Ronald's seizure, a mother in the radiation lounge asked me for Larry Allen's name so she could pray for him. Her son was taking radiation as an outpatient. He was her second son with a brain tumor, and his first sign of a tumor was a seizure. I could think of nothing else. Fear settled into my mind. Did Ronald also have a brain tumor? It was a terrible feeling to know that this was a possibility.

After two days of testing on Ronald, they wanted to run more tests; however, Ronald refused and checked himself out of the hospital. Ronald kept saying that if he had cancer, he'd never let the doctors do to him what he'd seen them do to his brother.

I was so worried.

Dr. Donohue and I talked, and he felt that Ronald's condition could be due to exhaustion and a poor diet. Ronald was working eight- to ten-hour days and spending nights at the hospital, eating only one meal a day.

April 1–10, 1986

I wanted Larry Allen to be moved home to Parkview Hospital in Fort Wayne, but the doctors said he isn't stable enough. His hemoglobin continues to drop. Dr. Donohue feels it is due to bone marrow problems from the chemotherapy, radiation treatments, and malnutrition.

No date has been scheduled for the brain surgery. Surgery was done on his kidneys, however, and afterward he suffered from bladder spasms. A triple lumen catheter came out and had to be replaced. His kidney tubes remained. Larry Allen is eating baby cereal today. His weight has dropped to 115.

He had his twenty-fourth and final radiation treatment on April 8. I gave him a good bath today and discussed moving him to Parkview Hospital. Larry Allen said it would be nicer there and that he could help Rod with his homework. The kidney doctor said it was fine that he be moved.

I feel our family members need to be in the same town and that Larry A. would feel better if he were closer to home. Stress is taking its toll on all of us; after all, it's been nine months, and we've all experienced a roller coaster of emotions. They say God won't give you more than you can handle—but I think we're getting to the breaking point. I feel so horrible about all the pain Larry Allen has been facing. No mother wants to see her son or family suffer this much.

Larry Allen feels he might need something for depression. We hugged and cried together. He is so tired of fighting this and being in the hospital. He wants to be well again. "How can the family take all this?" Larry Allen asked me. He worried about the rest of us. He is always so thoughtful.

"I think your depression is due to the fact that you're finally realizing just how sick you've been," I suggested.

"I want to go home," Larry Allen told me. "Not to the Fort Wayne hospital, but home."

Larry Allen desperately wants to be well again. He hates that his family is running back and forth, from home to the hospital. Dr. Corry seems to be dragging his feet on organizing Larry Allen's move. There seems to be some confusion over who is to make the arrangements.

Larry Allen slept better last night and was able to sit in a chair three times today. They cut back his food line, hoping this would increase his appetite.

April 11–15, 1986

I asked Dr. Corry why they'd put Larry Allen through testing to check for a leak or blockage if they planned to do nothing about the leak.

Larry Allen didn't sleep well last night. I suggested he try reading the next time he had trouble sleeping. They shut off his I.V. and told him to drink more on his own. I told them he would dehydrate. The dietitian came in with a calorie chart and explained how much he had to eat.

The test they ran showed blockage in the urethra tubes and a leak in the left urethra tube. Larry Allen is very upset; he cried when he heard the results. He wants to be out of the hospital. I explained to him that he can't eat, walk, or bath himself, but I think he feels that I don't want him to be home. I told him he's come too far to lose it all now. He cried and wouldn't talk to me. I felt so discouraged. I hate to tell him no.

His white blood count is high; he may be getting an infection due to poor nutrition. A spinal tap was done to remove fluid for testing. I told Dr. Corry that I was worried about his mental health. Dr. Corry said he has never seen anyone be so close to death and yet not die.

The doctors want to run more tests, but I hate to see Larry Allen go through it; he's in so much pain. I wish I could stop it. It hurts so much to see him suffer. When they put him on that hard table for tests, his pain increases. He weighs only 115 pounds. We decided that we are taking Larry Allen home on Monday, with or without the doctors' consent. I have asked the doctors to prepare his records for our departure.

Dr. Hozze came in to see him. He seems like a super doctor, and I wish he'd been on Larry Allen's case earlier. They are going to put him on an antidepressant. Larry Allen told Dr. Hozze that what bothered him the most is that each doctor, chief resident, or medical student tells him something different about his progress and when he'll be able to leave. Dr. Hozze told Larry Allen he'd ask the doctors to communicate among themselves and have one spokesperson.

Larry Allen told Dr. Hozze that he doesn't eat because he's never hungry. Dr. Hozze suggested hypnosis, and Larry Allen agreed to give it a try.

On April 14, Larry Allen's temperature was 98.6, his pulse was 124, and his blood pressure was 108 over 70. He's dehydrated and has lost twenty-five pounds since February 12. They did physical therapy on him today. Afterward, he was really tired and slept most of the day.

We asked Ronald to watch Larry Allen while we made the arrangements to move him to Parkview Hospital.

The doctors said Larry Allen was not stable enough to move and that Dr. Einhorn had to get in touch with Dr. Myers so he could be admitted to Parkview Hospital; the doctors wanted him to stay. One of the nurses helped us get Larry Allen ready to move. Once the doctors realized we were leaving with or without their consent, they were supportive and helped with the arrangements. One of the doctors said he'd do the same if it were his son.

We felt that Larry Allen's spirit had been broken in the I.C.U. and that it would be good for him to get away from the medical center. The center was not designed for long-term care, and he needed a different environment.

Dr. Foggon wanted to run more tests on Larry Allen before we departed, but Larry Allen said no.

A social worker came in and said the insurance would not pay for an ambulance unless there was a medical reason. Dr. Hozze said he'd fill out the papers and document that it was for Larry Allen's mental health.

It was raining hard when we finally left the medical center. This time, Larry Allen had been a patient there for a grand total of sixty-one days. We had paramedics go with Larry Allen; they kept him on an I.V. and Hyperale and gave him a shot of Darvocet for the pain. We arrived at Parkview Hospital at 7:20 PM. Dr. Nutom was on call that night and attended us in the emergency room. He asked me if I remembered him—I did. Unfortunately, we'd received poor care from Dr. Nutom early on in Larry Allen's case. I'd reported it to Dr. Myers and told him exactly what I thought concerning Dr. Nutom.

It felt good to be in Fort Wayne again, but it was hard to leave Ronald in Indy alone. When we left him at the medical center, he looked depressed. It has to be hard for Ronald to have the rest of the family in the same town while he's alone in Indy. For all these months, his life has been work and helping with Larry Allen. We need to give up the apartment and get Ronald moved back home; the family needs to be together.

Dr. Nutom could not do enough for Larry Allen. Immediately, he put Larry Allen in a small private room and said he'd move him to a larger, nicer room as soon as one was available. They treated him like a V.I.P.

The doctors at the I.U. Medical Center told us to contact Dr. Tryeer in Fort Wayne. We did so, and when Dr. Tryeer came in, he stood at Larry Allen's bedside and stared for some time. I asked about hypnosis as a way to treat his eating disorder, but he felt it wouldn't help. He asked Larry some questions and then went out of the room and wrote up orders for three different drugs. I told the nurse not to have them sent up, that Larry Allen would not be taking any of them. The nurse was glad I requested that the order be canceled. Drugs are not always the answer.

April 15, 1986

Dr. Nutom came in and checked Larry Allen's vital signs. He felt Larry Allen was dehydrated and had a case of hypertension. I asked about having Dr. Tryeer taken off Larry Allen's case. When Dr. Nutom asked why, I explained that we didn't feel that drugs would resolve Larry Allen's eating and appetite disorders. Dr. Nutom agreed and said he'd notify Dr. Tryeer.

One of the nurses told me she was in a doctor's conference that morning and they discussed Larry Allen. She said that the doctors are excited about being on his case. After hearing all the things they discussed, she felt that Larry Allen has to be a miracle and that God has a special purpose for him and the family.

April 16, 1986

Larry Allen slept restlessly, and he was disoriented today. He gets mixed up about where we are. Doctors say it's important to keep talking to him about daily things.

April 17, 1986

Dr. Drieer says that Larry Allen's HMG is too low; he'll need a blood transfusion soon. I hate that they use random blood here and not blood from our own donors. I worry about AIDS.

Dr. Drieer said it was an oversight that Dr. Rudolph had not been called in on the case. Later, Dr. Rudolph came in and seemed to be a super doctor. He trained under Dr. Donohue and calls him his boss. His sister is a nurse at the I.U. Medical Center.

Larry Allen started physical therapy in his room today.

Great news—he smiled for the first time in a very long while. He's on his way to getting well! Yeah!

April 18, 1986

Larry Allen has gained two pounds, but some of this is fluid retention. Dr. Drieer says the pneumonia is gone. He was given two units of blood.

April 19, 1986

Larry Allen slept well last night and ate a good breakfast. He walked to a chair. He seems a little grouchy today.

April 20, 1986

Larry Allen's heart rate at 1:00 AM went up to 208. Between 2:00 AM and 6:00 AM it averaged 140 to 160. An EKG was done at 6:00 AM and showed no problem. Dr. Myers and Dr. Nutom were called in. Dr. Nailsun felt Larry Allen's rise in heart rate was due to drugs. Dr. Nailsun wants Larry Allen to get two units of blood and packed cells. I think Dr. Nailsun is a good doctor.

April 21, 1986

Larry Allen ate well today, but he is depressed and bored. I suggested various things to do, but he refuses to do them. He was able to bathe and feed himself. His right ankle is causing him a lot of pain. They feel it could be a stress fracture caused by not walking for an extended period of time. He had physical and occupational therapy. He ate his supper sitting in a chair.

Larry Allen will not eat breakfast until I arrive at the hospital. As soon as Jason gets on the school bus, I head over. The rest of the family takes turns going to the hospital in the evenings. During my weeks at the I.U. Medical Center, I had only Larry Allen to concentrate on; now I feel more pressure to cope with the rest of the family's needs. I feel torn when I'm not at the hospital. Larry A. has suffered so much and has great faith. Larry Sr. and I feel so blessed that he's still alive.

April 22, 1986

The Hyperale was turned up today. I need to have a doctor's permission to look at Larry Allen's medical charts.

Physical therapy seems to be helping, but he is exhausted afterward.

One of Larry Allen's primary specialists said, "He is hanging on the edge of a cliff with one foot hanging over and the other foot on a banana peel." Right now he feels like the banana peel is under Larry Allen's foot, but he's steady. Sometimes when he's very sick, the specialist says, "I'm doing the electric slide on the banana peel."

April 23, 1986

Larry Allen's ankle is still hurting a lot. Dr. Datmer encouraged him to keep working with the physical therapist. I made Larry Allen wash himself again today for the added exercise. I told him that the more he can do for himself, the better he'd start to feel. I told him that before he could go home he'd need to be able to take care of himself.

Larry Allen does not like occupational therapy. He feels that it's stupid to type things. They have also asked me to encourage him to cut up his own meat. He doesn't like going down to physical therapy. He feels they make him wait around too long before bringing him back to his room. He's exhausted after his therapies. I go with him to therapy to make sure he doesn't have to wait for someone to bring him back to bed.

He was very quiet when I told him I had to meet Jason after school but that his dad would be up after he got off work. It's so hard to do anything that I feel might upset him; after all he's been through. But I knew he had to be encouraged to take care of himself again.

April 24, 1986

Larry Allen is tired and down today. He'll hardly talk to us. I asked him when he felt it was most important for someone to be at the hospital with him, and he said during meal times. I agree that this is the best time. He has such negative thoughts about food, and he has to reacquire a desire for it. All the vomiting and the long periods of not eating were enemies to his digestive system. Those weren't easy times—the possibility of throwing it all up, or the blotting, the pain it created as it passed through his body. Perhaps this is what he is thinking about at meal times.

April 25, 1986

Dr. Datmer changed the triple lumen tube. Larry Allen has a terrible scar where the medical center put it in. However, his spirits are much better today. He wants to leave the hospital for the opening day of Jason's Little League season. Dr. Datmer told him that would be fine as long as he stays hydrated.

April 26, 1986

Larry Allen's I.V. was turned off at 10:30 AM, and we left the hospital at 10:55 AM for the baseball game. It's hot outside, but the game only lasted for one hour. Due to the heat, Larry Allen dehydrated faster than usual, and he wanted to go home. He hadn't been out of the hospital for two and a half months. We all went home and ate pizza. Then he was ready to go back and get his I.V. hooked up. It felt great having all the family together at home.

April 27, 1986

Larry Allen is very tired today—yesterday wore him out. He didn't eat much, and he's so thin and weak. Being so limited at his age must be very upsetting for him. Before his illness, he was very ambitious and athletic.

April 28, 1986

Larry Allen is still feeling physically exhausted and is tired of being in the hospital. I tried to encourage him to find activities in the hospital to occupy his time: string art, puzzles, and reading. He has a large private room, so he can set up several activities.

The doctors also want him to consume two thousand calories a day. Larry Allen will agree to anything in order to get out of the hospital.

Later, he played two games of backgammon with his dad. It was like old times for them.

Larry Allen is able to feed and bathe himself again, and he weighs 123 pounds. He asked if I knew that he and his father had an argument last night about his not eating. I told him that I did know and that his father had hurt feelings. I explained that, as parents, we were trying to do everything possible to help him. It was important that he accepts his health limits and finds things to occupy his time until he regains his physical strength.

Dr. Donohue informed us that Larry Allen does not remember his physical struggles before the brain tumor.

May 4, 1986

Larry Allen weighs 126 pounds and had the I.V. taken off this afternoon. Salt from his kidneys is improving, but the doctors aren't sure if this is because of his medications or because his kidneys are getting better. On May 3, dehydration was a problem. On May 4, Dr. Rudolph removed the clamps from the outer kidney tubes. Larry Allen lost two pounds because the food line was off and he was grouchy and depressed. He told us he couldn't handle more setbacks, such as another tumor or some other physical shutdown.

I feel that Larry Allen is literally a survivor. I'm so proud of how hard he's working to get home. The challenge for him is for his body to survive the chemo, radiation, and surgeries. I think getting out of hospital and back at home with his family would be a great healer.

May 5, 1986

Larry Allen is begging to go home, so they went ahead and released him. His balance is extremely poor, and during the night he fell forward off the toilet. I'm afraid he might eventually hurt himself badly. His appetite is poor, but he is still trying to eat. He slept all afternoon but sat on the porch for about forty-five minutes when Jason came home from school.

The family feels blessed and thankful that he's made it home. I know being in a home setting will help his recovery.

He's a fighter and a survivor! Thank you, Jesus!

May 15, 1986

Larry Allen was dehydrated, so he was admitted to the hospital and hooked up to I.V. fluids. We arrived home from Parkview after spending several days on I.V. fluids. Larry Allen looks much better, and he really needed the fluids.

May 23, 1986

Larry Allen is depressed today and dehydrated from losing salt. A chemical imbalance or his electrolytes could be the cause. The doctor isn't sure. Each setback is stressful for him—and there is always the worry that the cancer will reappear.

May 29, 1986

Larry Allen was given two units of blood at the oncology center, which helped him feel better and less dizzy. Fort Wayne will not allow us to use our own donors as Indy does. I have real concerns about random blood.

June 2, 1986

Larry A. weighs 117 pounds. Dizziness started yesterday, but he didn't tell anyone. He said he has a goal to eat two thousand calories a day. This is the first time he's set any goals since being sick—it's a good sign. He has been getting in the pool daily to regain his strength.

June 3, 1986

Frequent urination, some burning, and a swollen face. Dr. Drieer had Larry Allen take a urine culture to Parkview and ordered medication. Dr. Nailsun saw him in the office, and his blood pressure was low.

June 10, 1986

Larry Allen has gained three pounds. Dr. Nailsun feels we need to have his knee checked by an orthopedic doctor to see if he tore ligaments when he fell on May 27.

June 23, 1986

I took Larry Allen to Parkview for two X rays of his head and a CAT scan with contrast of his head. The family and I are stressed about the results, which will determine if he needs brain surgery.

June 24, 1986

When I called today, the test results were in, so I went to pick them up. Dr. Rudolph informed us that Larry Allen's CAT scan shows no sign of a brain tumor—only scar tissue. If one does begin to grow, he'd need to have surgery. Larry Allen would not be able to withstand any more radiation. I was so excited about the results. It was gamble to have them stop the chemo. After one round, the chemo was destroying his organs and making him sicker. The doctors told me that no one is sure how much chemo reaches the head area. Radiation would focus on the tumor.

Thank God; it's a miracle. I will take the results along to doctors' appointments at the medical center.

June 30, 1986

Dr. Donohue feels good about the CAT scan results but wants Larry Allen to be observed closely. The CAT scan does not show if it's scar tissue or a tumor starting up. The only sure way to know is to have a neurological surgeon open a flap at the site of tumor and check it out. We were told that Larry Allen's type of cancer is teratoma, which is the best type of malignancy to have. Some other types spread faster. The doctor suggested we have a CAT scan done every three months, and regular HCG blood tests and chest X rays for one year. The radiologist feels there would be more damage to the brain to remove scar tissue or calcium. Dr. Einhorn says calcium will disappear in time at the tumor site. He feels no more chemo is needed. He told Larry Allen not to return to work until he feels stronger, but he can start driving short distances.

July 1, 1986

I could tell Larry Allen is tired and has no appetite. I thought maybe it was from going to Indy and meeting with so many doctors. His side is full of pus and leaks. This is the area where the shunt site was unable to be stitched. I think Dr. Brucker, our plastic surgeon, should look at it.

July 14, 1986

We arrived at Parkview Hospital for surgery to remove the stint and check for leaks. Our son Rod was to have back surgery today for a ruptured disc. He and Larry Allen were in pre-op together. They came and took Rod to surgery. They gave Larry Allen a shot of Demerol and reran lab work. Dr. Rudolph came and told us his potassium is too low for anesthesia. Low potassium will cause heart problems during surgery. He was put on potassium pills, and they will recheck his levels in a week. They brought Rod to recovery; he'll be in the hospital for a few days. They won't do Larry Allen's surgery until after his party on July 26. We are having a party to celebrate his life and thank everyone who has helped and been supportive these past two years.

The church and school have been supportive by providing blood donations and fixing meals.

August 19, 1986

Larry Allen's weight is up to 134—he's gained nine pounds in six weeks. Rod and Larry Allen flew to the Bahamas for the day. They went to the casinos and had a great time. Several nurses and a friend of mine were on the trip, so I knew he was in good hands. Rod would watch him closely. They looked so happy and excited when they left. Larry Allen was tired when he returned, but he had a great day! God knows he needed some fun.

August 20, 1986

Larry Allen experienced a lot of vomiting, as well as pain on the left side and around the tailbone. It hurts for him to walk. Tubes were put in the urethra to help his urine output. The doctors feel that peeling the tumors off that area has caused poor blood supply. If the stints and dilation don't work, they may need to do reconstructive surgery on the tubes.

When most of Larry Allen's hair failed to grow back, the doctors felt it was due to the cobalt treatments. I was very upset about this. I'd specifically asked if it would do permanent damage. Should I trust anything they say?

Chapter 11

✦

Surgery

Told by Delila, Larry Allen's mother

September 1986

Larry Allen is planning on returning to work in November. He is experiencing headaches and vomiting, as well as side pain due to a swollen kidney. They took him to surgery, and Dr. Hamton said his stents were out of place and the tubes were completely blocked. His blood pressure is high: 180 over 120.

Dr. Nailsun talked with me about Larry's kidney diagnosis. I was upset about this setback, and I wasn't sure how Larry A. would cope with more bad news. He's worked so hard to recover, and this will be a major setback. We all feel like the roller coaster of life is headed downward again. His body has been through so much, and we worry about how much more he can physically handle.

Dr. Donohue called Larry A. and told him to come back to the I.U. Medical Center so he could figure out how to repair the urethra tubes. Larry A. trusts and respects him. He is a great Christian surgeon.

Scar tissue has formed at the leak sites. In four weeks they'll replace the large stent with a smaller one and use a balloon stent to stretch the tubes.

October 1986

Larry Allen is still having problems with vomiting, he feels really tired, and he's lost five pounds. His temperature is normal, and he is acting more alert, but he seems angry and will hardly talk to any of us. I'm sure he is very depressed. His surgery is planned for October 31. Dr. Donohue told us that the surgery will take most of the day and that he's never done this type of surgery on a patient who's had lymph node dissection. After the surgery, Larry Allen will remain in the I.C.U. for several days and in the hospital for two weeks.

October 31, 1986

We were all worried about the surgery. Larry A. is running a temperature, and his blood pressure is low. He looks very rundown. We wanted to postpone the surgery, but Larry wanted to go ahead with it.

At around 5:30 AM, we all arrived at the hospital. They gave Larry a pre-op shot at 6:30 AM to make him sleepy. They took him to the pre-op waiting area. We walked beside his gurney to the surgery doors. I felt that I couldn't handle leaving him once again at the double doors to go into surgery. The family went to the chapel to pray for a successful surgery. At 8:25 AM, a nurse reported that Larry's surgery was in progress. At 10:00 AM, they started working on the urethra tubes; at 12:00 PM, Nurse Gretchen reported that both tubes were very constricted, and the doctors were deciding what to do. Once reconstruction was underway, the surgery would go faster. Gretchen reported at 2:30 PM that they were working on bowel resection. The right side was complete at 4:30 PM, and they started on the left side. Larry was doing fine. When I went down to the cafeteria for coffee, I heard the interns talking about the Woodruff surgery that was still going on. It was the talk of the hospital, and in a hospital like this you don't want to be the topic of conversation—they deal with a lot of really bad stuff.

The surgery lasted eleven hours. Both urethra tubes were replaced by using the small intestines. The blood supply was good. The doctors feel that the surgery was successful, considering all of Larry Allen's problems. They moved him to the I.C.U. at 8:30 PM. He is off the respirator now, and his vital signs are good. We were able to see Larry at 9:15 PM. He looked swollen but is doing well. The surgery lounge was empty except for our family. Susan brought in pizza and soft drinks for our supper. Jason was sick with bronchitis all day and could hardly talk.

November 1, 1986

Larry Sr. and Rod arrived at the hospital at 6:30 AM to see Larry for a few minutes. He was asleep but looked good. The nurse said his vital signs were normal. He was taken off the oxygen. At noon they moved him to a room, which will allow us to be with him more. He walked from the hallway to his bed. They hooked him up to a morphine pump, which gives him 1.0 milligram every ten minutes for pain. There are seven tubes coming out of him.

Most days he feels tired and edgy; low blood pressure is usually the cause. Dr. Donohue feels that Larry is doing well, but problems with pain and nausea are a constant battle.

November 6, 1986

When the nurses removed Larry Allen from his bed to change his sheets, he became very nauseated. The doctor heard some bowel sounds. Larry Allen didn't talk much today; his voice is very weak. They check his blood sugar daily by pricking his finger. They put a bladder catheter in, and it will need to remain there for three to four days in order for the bladder to seal itself.

November 7, 1986

Today Larry Allen had the dry heaves. The doctor said that due to the extensive surgeries, it might take a while for Larry's bowels to function properly.

Rod gave him a bath today, and they started a new I.V. with Demerol for pain. The staples are to be removed from the stomach area today. Larry Allen wants to start the morphine pump, but he has to wait until the Demerol wears off.

November 10, 1986

Larry vomited more today, so they hooked up the stomach tubes. One of the nurses said that vomiting would occur when the tube is turned off because nothing can pass through to him. They worked with the tube for some time before it began to work properly. Larry may need to go home with the stomach tube hooked up. The nurse said she would talk with the doctor. She feels Larry is dehydrated. He still gets dizzy when he is up. He is also taking shots for nausea. His pulse is a little fast today.

The doctor is not concerned yet about the stomach problems. He said Larry could go home when he's able to eat but that we need to take it slowly.

November11, 1986

Larry Allen is craving Popsicles today and is not dizzy. He walked the floor twice and drank some lemon lime drink. The stomach tube is still hooked up, but he feels much better. Dr. Faster said he talked to Dr. Donohue on the phone, and Dr. Donohue said Larry could not be released until he's back in town and can check him over.

November 12, 1986

Larry Allen was in X ray for one hour and thirty minutes and seemed a little confused this morning, but he has not taken any morphine. His skin feels dry, but he's very thirsty. Dr. Donohue thinks they clamped the stomach tube off too soon, so he wants to run a stomach test before they clamp it off again.

November 13, 1986
Larry Allen seems to feel good today. He was able to sit in a chair for about an hour. There will be tests over the next several days to check for kidney leakage. If there are no leaks, they will remove the bags.

November 14, 1986
They started pulling the penrose drainage tube from Larry Allen's side, and the bladder didn't leak with the catheter out. His bowels seem to be working.

It was a very noisy night, and Larry Allen couldn't get much sleep. He had X rays and tests all day. The tests caused him to have diarrhea, but this is a good sign that things are getting through his system.

November 15, 1986
Three stomach bags were removed, and Larry Allen was given clear liquids. If he does okay, they'll try solids on Sunday. He did well when he walked to the lounge and sat for a while.

November 16, 1986
The doctor said Larry Allen should follow a regular diet today, and, if all goes well, he can go home on Monday. Around 5:00 PM, they turned off the Hyperale food line. Dr. Donohue is unsure if the new urethra tubes he made out of Larry's bowels will release enough urine. He said he'd know in about six months if the tubes were working properly.

November 17, 1986
Larry Allen must measure all urine output and work on caloric intake. His blood pressure is to be taken daily.

November 20, 1986

Larry Allen's appetite was poor, so he started drinking Ensure. His blood pressure dropped to 80/58. They feel this is due to dehydration or that his hemoglobin is too low from malnutrition. His voice is weak, and he is tired. He will be given two units of blood on Friday at Parkview Hospital. One of his tubes started to leak, and he is down to 120 pounds.

November 24, 1986

I took Larry Allen to see Dr. Donohue in Indianapolis, and they removed the gastric tube. The doctor said that low blood pressure means blood volume is down, and high blood pressure means he'd have a kidney problem, so low is better than high. The doctor wants to increase his calories and work on his nutrition.

December 4, 1986

Dr. Nailsun saw Larry today, and he weighed in at 128 pounds with a blood pressure of 100/78. The incision areas are all healing well. The septra medicine could cause thirst, so the doctor cut it in half. Larry Allen's urine output was good. The doctor does not recommend that he take flu shots.

December 10, 1986

Dr. Rudolph saw Larry Allen today. He weighed in at almost 129 and has normal HCG with no kidney infection. The doctor advised Larry Allen that if he ever goes to the emergency room to tell the doctors that his urethra tubes are made from his small intestines. Otherwise, they'll think he has a bad infection. The doctor wants Larry Allen to take in as many calories as possible and try a wide variety of foods.

December 22, 1986

Larry Allen saw Dr. Donohue today. The doctor feels the tubes are working well because of the level of creatine in the urine and urine output. Larry Allen can exercise more, but he must avoid bench pressing because it would be too hard on his stomach muscles. Dr. Donohue thinks Larry Allen is a miracle. Of course, we believe it's nothing short of a miracle that he' still with us. The doctor wishes the lymph node dissection had been done after the brain tumor. Cancer can lay dormant in the body for up to five years and then take off again.

January 6, 1987

Larry Allen weighed in at 136. Yeah! He flew to Florida with Grandpa Woodruff to visit his Uncle Wes and Aunt Peg. Their family had a birthday party for him during his visit. Grandpa was so happy that he could take this trip with Larry Allen.

February 1, 1987

Larry moved to Fall Creek Apartments in Indy. He still tires easily but is planning to work half days at the Hook Drugs corporate office. It is so hard for the family to leave him in Indy. He's worked so hard to survive and return to work. I'm so proud of him. We talk on the phone daily and see him on weekends.

February 3, 1987

This is milestone month for Larry Allen: he is able to return to work at Hook Drugs. Everyone there made him feel welcome, and they were all very glad to see him. Larry has been off work for eighteen months. Although he was tired and thin at the beginning, he was so happy to be alive. Larry Allen finds it lonely living alone. He's used to the family being around.

The company he worked for was always supportive and cooperative. The insurance was good and gave us the option of having the best doctors and private rooms. Larry Allen pushes himself to regain his strength and energy level. His body has been through so much with fighting the cancer with chemo and radiation. The family goes to Indy on weekends to spend time with him. What a blessing.

March 9, 1987

I go with Larry Allen for his checkups. Dr. Donohue feels he is doing remarkably well with the new tubes. He wants to have a CAT scan done before our next visit. Larry Allen will go back for a checkup on August 20. Dr. Donohue reminded us that the cancer is still the number-one problem and that Larry Allen must be watched closely. Larry Allen has no memory of part of his illness. Dr. Donohue told us that is how the mind protects us when we are critically ill. It's a great blessing for Larry Allen. I wish our family had no memory of the critical times and suffering we've watched our son and brother go through. I heard the noise of the life support machines for months, long after Larry Allen had been off them.

April 1987

I see all the positive changes in Larry Allen's life. He's adjusted to being back on his own. He enjoys being back to work on computers. This is what he went to Purdue to learn. He has a great support system of coworkers; they've been so supportive. Larry Allen is working on muscle strength. Being in bed all those months made them weak.

May 1987

The family and I are always thankful to see Larry Allen. On alternate weekends, he comes home. It takes your breath away to watch Larry Allen and his brothers shoot hoops and laugh together. We never tire of watching all five of our sons having fun. I look at all of this as a miracle. I pray that Larry Allen never has any future suffering or pain. The family has seen him at death's door so many times in the past two years. We are so thankful that the family worked together to get through this. I'm sure that each of us knows Larry Allen would do the same for any of us. Each time Larry Allen went to surgery, the family went to the chapel to pray for his safety. Thank you, God, for allowing us to keep him longer.

June 17, 1987

The chest X ray and blood test came back with no trace of cancer! It's a miracle that Larry Allen made it through this. Thank you, Jesus!

Larry A. had to make some adjustments to living alone again. Rod postponed college for a semester to help care for Larry Allen during his illness. Ronald helped pay for Larry Allen's apartment and bills in Indy, and he also helped us care for him. Donald helped at home by keeping an eye on Jason. Many times, Jason stayed all night at the hospital and had to spend a lot of time entertaining himself. Jason struggled with the many changes in his young life. He always looked up to his big brother, Larry Allen, and I think he had a great fear of losing him.

It's nothing but a miracle that he is still with us and back into the swing of life. I worry a lot about a recurrence of the cancer; when he experiences any headaches or is not feeling well, he, too, begins to worry. Many tell us that Larry Allen is an inspiration. They share their own battles with cancer, and Larry Allen gives them hope.

During the past two years, we formed several close relationships with other young men fighting cancer. One by one, they died over the years. Each time Larry Sr. and I went to the funeral home, we fearfully thought that our son could be next. We grieved with the families who had fought so hard with their loved ones and lost.

We will always want to protect Larry Allen from pain. We feel he has experienced more pain than most people do in their lifetimes. Each time we look at him, we're reminded of the miracle God gave us: life.

PART III

EXCERPTS FROM OUR JOURNALS

Haven't I commanded you: be strong and courageous?
Do not be afraid or discouraged,
for the Lord your God is with you wherever you go.

Joshua 1:9

Chapter 12

✦

The Interview

Told by Delila, Larry Allen's mother

I had been told at the I.U. Medical Center that they questioned the environment in New Haven because of the number of cancer patients from that area. That got me thinking about the environment, so I contacted a local cancer society. When we were in town, we attended and led some support groups there. The participants shared their concerns with me. I asked myself if we could be living in cancer cluster. I felt morally obligated to contact the media to have them look into this. I knew the agony of watching someone suffer with cancer, and I hoped I could help save even one other person from experiencing it. It can take ten to twenty years for cancer to develop after toxic exposure.

After the media released their concerns, some area residents were concerned only about property value. I struggled to fathom how anyone could compare property values with precious life. After I contacted the media, I agreed to an appointment for an interview with Larry Allen and me.

✶✶✶✶

On the day of the interview, I opened the door. A woman greeted me with a smile and a handshake. "Hello—I'm Amy from the local news. Are you Delila?"

"Yes. Please come in, Amy." I stood aside, and Amy walked into the foyer carrying a burgundy leather briefcase. She followed me into the formal living area, where I offered her a seat.

"Can I get you anything to drink?" I asked.

"No, thank you. I'm fine."

Amy bent down and opened her briefcase; her curly brown hair fell forward. She was elegantly petite, dressed smartly in a fitted navy skirt and white blouse. She took out a file as I sat on the sofa across from her.

"As you know," Amy began, "we've learned of Larry Allen's struggle with cancer through the Cancer Society. Obviously, he is not the only one in this area fighting the disease. Did I understand you correctly when you told me over the phone that several of Larry Allen's schoolmates and friends came down with cancer?"

"Yes, but Larry Allen is the only survivor."

Amy said nothing; tears formed in my eyes. I knew that the families whose sons died from cancer at such a young age would be the hardest to interview. Even though Larry Allen beat the cancer, what physical problems would he face as a result of his treatments? What irreparable damage had already been done?

"I have a list of questions here that we'll ask you and Larry Allen during the TV interview." Amy handed the paper to me. "You can look them over, and then, in about a week we'll set up a time to do the live interview."

"Will we need to come down to the TV station?"

"Actually, I think it would work well if we did the interview here in your living room. Would that be okay with you?"

"Yes, that's fine," I agreed.

Larry Allen came into the room. Although he was still very thin and pale from his ordeal, his smile seemed to brighten the room.

"Hi, I'm Larry Allen," he said, taking a seat next to me.

"It's good to meet you, Larry. I'm Amy from the local news. Thank you for helping us with this interview."

"I'm happy to help."

"What we have learned about all of this is quite shocking," Amy told us. "And I think we've only begun to touch the surface of this problem. I still have an environmentalist and a toxicologist to interview before we proceed. I gave your mother a list of questions that we'll most likely ask during the interview. However, I'm sure we'll add a few more before the actual shoot. I'll let you know about the added questions beforehand so you can think about how best to answer them." She paused for a moment. "Do you have any questions?"

"You will keep us informed about what you learn concerning the area?" I asked.

"Oh, yes," Amy said, nodding. "We won't withhold any information. There are times I think that's my true calling: to inform the public. And when I inform the public, I want to give them the truth of the matter. As Americans, we deserve that much."

Amy stood with her briefcase in hand. "Well, I have several other families to talk with, so I must be on my way."

Larry Allen and I stood.

"Thank you both for taking the time to do this. I feel it's important to get the word out."

"It is important," I told her. "I just wish it could have been brought to light many years ago, before our children had to suffer."

Amy's mouth twisted slightly, and her hazel eyes became compassionate. "I wish that, too. Unfortunately, tragedy usually strikes before anything is ever done about a problem."

"Yes, it seems that way," I agreed.

Amy left to interview other families in the area. Larry Allen and I went into the dining area and sat down to look over the information Amy gave us concerning the upcoming interview. A list of questions and what to expect during the shoot were outlined.

"We need to think each question over and be ready to give the best answer," I said. "This is too important not to."

"What do you think they'll uncover during these interviews and investigations?" Larry Allen asked.

"Who knows?"

"It's almost frightening to think of the possibilities. Think about it, Mom: it's possible that we've all been exposed to whatever it is they feel has caused this cancer."

I sighed heavily. "Yes, it's crossed my mind, but I try not to think about it. I just couldn't bear to see another one of my boys suffer what you went through." I thought about Larry Allen telling me that he prayed that none of his brothers would be faced with the same fate that befell him.

February 4, 1987: Local TV News Report

"Poison Playgrounds," the title of the report, was shot in the Meadowbrook subdivision of New Haven, Indiana. Amy began her interview standing next to the Meadowbrook School playground. Microphone in hand, she explained, "The many residents of the Meadowbrook subdivision became alarmed when many young people from this area were diagnosed with cancer. This prompted the residents to call the Cancer Society and ask that they take note of the number of young people who have developed cancer in their area." Amy paused for a moment and then bravely and boldly spoke out. "Is it possible that the heavy industry in the New Haven area could be the cause of all the health problems? The Meadowbrook Association has claimed that industrial companies are burning uranium late at night and dumping leaded paint into the river. Many people are taking a hard look at the environment, and some believe contamination is coming from the creek that snakes its way through the Meadowbrook subdivision. Could the hazardous waste that was burned and buried in the 1950s and 1960s be the cause of many of the victims' cancers? Unfortunately," she went on, "there's probably no way to determine the health effects the waste has caused."

The cameraman gave a panoramic view of the playground and then refocused on Amy. She continued, "Kevin Donley died last June. Kevin's death and Larry Allen Woodruff's struggle with cancer have alarmed the people living in the Meadowbrook subdivision." Amy turned, and the camera zoomed in on her as the live broadcast continued.

"Larry Allen Woodruff, age twenty-four, has been battling cancer for one and a half years, and his struggle continues. He, along with many of his friends, grew up in the Meadowbrook subdivision area and played on the same playgrounds. Many families in the neighborhood were touched by cancer and were treated at the same hospital. Several, however, were treated at a cancer center in Texas. The Cancer Society has determined that this is a cluster area for cancer. Not only is it very unusual for eighteen- and nineteen-year-olds to be diagnosed with cancer, but also these teens are from the same area. There are many whole families from New Haven who have very serious health problems. We feel that it is worthy to continue these investigations, and we hope to get a response from the State Board of Health."

The next interview was done at our home. Larry Allen and I sat on the sofa during the interview. Amy began by explaining the previous broadcast. "Is it possible," she began, "that hazardous waste, such as the burning of uranium late at night and the dumping of leaded paint in the rivers, could be the cause of many fatal illnesses and serious health problems for people in the Meadowbrook area? I'm here in the home of Larry and Delila Woodruff, who had been residents of Meadowbrook. Their son, Larry Allen Woodruff, along with many of their neighbors, has battled cancer. Many of the residents feel that the hazardous waste and lethal chemicals are the causes of their health problems." Amy then asked Larry Allen how he felt about living in a toxic area.

"It's sad," Larry Allen stated, "that this happened so many years ago, and now we have to pay the price."

"How do you feel about all of this, Delila?" Amy asked.

"Our goal today is to prevent other families from going through what many of the families have had to face in the Meadowbrook area."

Amy continued, "We have discussed the problems with the Board of Health, and they have stated that the area's problem is worth looking into. However, there aren't enough funds to proceed. I've talked with many residents who have said they'll do whatever it takes to get the problem in their area looked into.

"How can you protect your family from environmental effects? The Board of Health suggests that before you buy or build a home, have the soil tested. We will never know the extent of this problem. I believe it is a matter of grave concern for many of us. What can we do, as American citizens, to stop our environment from becoming toxic and our playgrounds poisoned?"

The interview was over, and Amy let out a heavy sigh.

Bill, her cameraman, gave her a thumbs-up. "You did it again," he reassured her. "It went great."

Amy raised her eyebrows and handed him the microphone. "Well, let's just hope we don't have too much negative feedback."

"Everyone needs to know about this," he assured her.

Amy thanked us for our participation.

Little did Amy know that the interviews and the exposé would cost her her job. Unbeknownst to many people, she was fired from her position with the local news. The next broadcast with a different newsperson went something like this:

"We feel that much of the blame was misplaced. It's not the big corporation that could be the cause of our hazardous waste problems. The truth is that it's much closer to home than we think. The consumer products that we throw into our trash are putting us in danger. Oven cleaners, paints, scouring powders—all of this can cause skin and eye damage.

"The Board of Health says that these materials contain solvents. Breathing these solvents for the long term can cause serious health problems. Weed killer is similar to Agent Orange. Dumping these products into our landfills is causing our hazardous waste problems. Yes, it is you and I who have caused our health issues. We must therefore blame ourselves for what we have done to the environment."

Soon forgotten was the fact that a local industrial company dumped massive amounts of chemicals and burned hazardous waste. The blame, as many see it, was truly misplaced, from the original source to the victims. How can the minority fight against the industry? How can so few people, with limited incomes, fight against the wealthy and powerful? All hope was gone for our small community, and Larry Allen's fight to live would continue for the remainder of his forty-one years on this earth.

Life is precious and can so easily be affected by our consumption and contamination of the environment. We cannot take back time or its effects, but we can change the future for our children. We can learn from our mistakes and change what causes disease and destroys life. The future is in our hands, and it is up to us to make that difference.

Chapter 13

◆

A Wife's Thoughts

Told by Kim, Larry Allen's wife

Larry A. and I started our lives together in 1987. I was going through a divorce and had a ten-month-old baby. He was cancer-free, just starting to live a normal life. We got married in 1988 and started our lives together in Indianapolis. Things were going well until his attacks started, which included aphasia, numbness, blurred vision, and headaches, around 1995. The attacks were short and had no lasting effects, but we couldn't figure out what was causing them. Life went on as usual until July 1996. The weekend we moved into our brand-new house, he had an attack that took us to the emergency room. He came out of it okay and continued working, but the doctors started running more tests.

A month later, during Labor Day weekend, he came home from work with a headache. We were celebrating our son's tenth birthday; he was having a sleepover at the house. Larry A. went to bed, and things were never the same again. He ended up in the hospital, and the seizures started; he was sent to intensive care and was put on a ventilator. He spent weeks in the hospital, and then he had to go through a complete rehabilitation program. We went through this many times over the next eight years.

Life was very hard for Larry A., but you never once heard him complain. He was always a joy to be around. Family and sports always meant a lot to him. Every time he went through rehab, one of the most important things for him to learn to do was read the newspaper so he would know when his games were on. He also really liked to chew tobacco—he'd find ways to buy it without my knowing, such as crossing a busy street to go to a gas station. He'd do this while he was going through rehab.

During those eight years, Larry A. was never able to return to his job due to his brain injury. However, working and driving were very important to him. He was able to get his driver's license renewed, and he drove locally. He worked as a volunteer at the hospital; he really enjoyed being around people and helping them. I'll never forget the time when he was living at a rehabilitation center and I went to pick him up, finding him still in a wheelchair but trying to help the other patients. He always thought of others first.

Life for the boys was very hard. They lost their dad when the attacks changed him permanently. They were six and ten. The dad they knew now wasn't the same; they had to help look out for him. We constantly looked for signs for when the next attack would hit. Many times, he'd go to yell at one of the boys and yell at the wrong one; or, when he'd go to correct them, he'd have the situation wrong. All of these things were caused by his brain injury. It was also a struggle for him to help out around the house. Many times he felt helpless. We always tried to make sure he got plenty of rest and didn't overdo it. When he got tired, he wasn't able to think as well.

Despite all of his ups and downs, Larry A. always made the most out of life. He was a very happy person, and he very rarely let things get him down. I'll never forget his last Thanksgiving, when he was out on a pass from rehab. We were sitting at the table eating when he started crying, wondering what he was doing wrong and why he kept getting sick. It broke all of our hearts to see him like that. We tried to convince him that it was nothing he did. We all loved him so much and would have done anything to take his pain away.

Now I think of Larry A. as my guardian angel. I know he's up there looking out for us. Life without Larry A. is very different. We all spent so many years looking out for him, talking to doctors, and trying to figure out what was causing the attacks. It was always so hard to watch him struggle. After each coma, he fought so hard to walk and talk—and then he'd get knocked down again. However, he never lost his determination to live. He will always be loved and never forgotten. He taught all of us many things about life and what is important.

Epilogue

Worry is wasting today's time to clutter up tomorrow's
opportunities with yesterday's trouble.

Told by Larry Sr., Larry Allen's father

June 1987

Kim Showman came over to visit the family and have us
meet her ten-month-old son, Blaine, from a previous marriage.
Our families had camped together when Larry A. and Kim
were teenagers. They dated a couple of times in high school.
Larry A. was home for a weekend visit; he and Kim picked up
where they left off and started dating again. Larry A. fell in
love with Kim and Blaine, and it was a great relationship for
both of them.

February 7, 1988

Today is Larry A.'s birthday. He's been cancer-free for
two years. He proposed to Kim, and she accepted. It was like
watching the pieces of his life come together. We felt blessed
that his life was starting to work out.

August 13, 1988

Larry A. and Kim were married at Emanuel Lutheran
Church in New Haven. It was a beautiful wedding. Larry A.'s
four brothers and his cousin Brad were the groomsmen. Blaine
was the ring bearer. Grandma Beth is ninety-two years old,
and Delila's sister Carlyne brought her for this blessed day.

Larry Allen and Kim took a honeymoon cruise. Later on, Larry Allen took guardianship of Blaine and had Blaine's last name changed to Woodruff. Larry Allen continues to work at Hook Drugs as a programmer/analyst, and Kim teaches special ed.

June 1989

Larry Allen and Kim built their first house and are expecting a baby. It's like Larry A. is finally getting to live his life and put the illness behind him. Each year that he stays cancer-free is a great sign.

May 14, 1990

Kim called us in Fort Wayne to tell us she was in labor. They planned to take Blaine to a sitter and then go to the hospital. We left for Indy, and guess what—we arrived at the hospital a few minutes before they did. They were blessed with a son and named him Jeremy.

I think this was the happiest day of Larry Allen's life. I'm so thankful we could be there for the great event. Larry A. feels blessed to have two sons.

Highlights of the Next Six Years of Larry Allen's Life

This was great time in Larry Allen's life.

Jeremy took his first steps.

He played on a men's softball team.

He coached Blaine's Little League team.

He attended church at Trinity Lutheran and served as an elder.

He watched Blaine start kindergarten at Trinity Lutheran.

His parents moved to Indianapolis and were able to spend more time with him and his family.

He went to work for the same computer-consulting firm where his dad worked.

Jeremy started preschool at Trinity Lutheran, which Delila taught.

There were swimming and cookouts at our house, with his brothers, Kim, and the boys.

He spoke at Cancer Survivor Day in Indianapolis.

He visited other young men in the hospital who were dealing with cancer and offered them his faith and encouragement.

He vacationed with Kim, Blaine, and Jeremy in the summer.

August 1, 1996

Larry A. and Kim had a new, bigger house built for them in an upstart neighborhood. Today is moving day. I was watching Jeremy at our house when he hit his head on the side of our swimming pool and had to be taken to a local hospital for stitches. Larry Allen had a migraine that night after moving. He'd had a few before, and the doctor said it was a complex migraine. It had been a stressful day, so we thought that's what had caused it.

August 30, 1996

This was Blaine's birthday, and he had friends over to spend the night. Larry Allen came home from work with a headache, vomiting, left-side numbness, and prolonged confusion.

He went to bed, thinking it was bad migraine and would be better tomorrow. Grandma Knapp helped watch the grandchildren the next day when his condition had worsened and he was admitted to the I.U. Medical Center. Doctors believed it could have been a stroke, but the test didn't confirm it. He started having seizures and was in put a semi coma state in the I.C.U. in order to stop the seizures. After a week, they brought him out of the coma. The seizures had stopped; he was left with action tremors, paralysis on one side, and cognitive impairment. The doctors had no idea what caused this attack.

Larry A. was upset and concerned about not being able to be the father he wants to be for Blaine and Jeremy. He is frustrated by tremors and paralysis. He had been active at his church, Trinity Lutheran. Pastor Herfurth showed his support through prayers and visits.

Larry Allen's recovery over the next several weeks was very slow. He worked hard to regain his skills. On Fridays, I took him to rehab and observed his progress. We would go to breakfast first, trying to make it a special time. I was so proud of how hard he worked and the nice comments the therapists made about his determination and positive attitude. The rehab doctor was amazed by his improvements. He was left with an action tremor on his left hand and arm and cognitive impairment.

October 1996 (Told by Delila, Larry Allen's mother)
Because the local doctors didn't know what was causing Larry Allen's attacks and we knew it wasn't a stroke, we went to the Mayo Clinic for a diagnosis. Larry A. wanted to know if he would have another brain attack. Kim, Larry Sr., Rod, and I took a week's vacation to help take Larry A. to the Mayo Clinic in Rochester, Minnesota.

The doctor in charge of Larry A.'s case said the delayed effects of the long-term radiation used on the brain tumor caused the attacks. Most patients didn't survive as long as Larry A., and doctors were only now starting to see how long-term radiation affected patients. The doctors ran daily tests to confirm this diagnosis. The only test the doctors wanted but did not do right away was an angiography[9]; that would wait until next week.   I told the doctor that Larry A. was sensitive and allergic to dyes, but he assured me that they rarely saw any reaction. We scheduled the angiography for the next Monday. Larry A. wanted to go home and see his boys, so we went home with the idea of going back to Mayo the Sunday before his scheduled test. Larry A. spent the weekend playing

---

9   Angiography: the radiographic visualization of the blood vessels after injection of a radiopaque substance (dye).

with his boys. When it was time to go back, Larry A. said he'd rather not go back, but he knew he should in order to see if they could stop the attacks. The test was to be done on an outpatient basis, and we would be gone one night. Ronald and I took him back to Mayo.

The angiography showed no problem, but Larry had an allergic reaction to the dye; within hours he developed aphasia, mental confusion, tremors, headache, poor vision, vomiting, and seizures. He was admitted to the hospital. Ronald and I took a week off work and stayed at Mayo to help. Larry Sr. and Kim traveled to the clinic that weekend, about 550 miles. I'm so upset that we went back for this test; the doctor said he had an allergic reaction to the dye, just as I'd feared. They couldn't get the seizures under control. Kim and I stayed there and worked on getting him moved to the I.U. Medical Center in Indy.

Three weeks later, Larry Allen was stable enough to be flown back to the I.U. Medical Center; Larry Allen, Kim, and I were flown back by air ambulance. Larry Sr. and an ambulance met us at the airport, ready to transfer Larry Allen to the hospital. When we landed, Larry A. had a seizure and was given a shot. Larry Sr. wondered why we weren't getting off the plane. At the I.U. Medical Center, Larry Allen was put into a drug-induced coma to stop the seizures.

Larry Sr. had been watching Blaine and Jeremy while Kim and I were at Mayo. The boys were so worried and stressed. They asked me the next day, "Is our dad going to die?" I held back the tears as I answered them: "We're not sure." They need to pray hard for his survival.

December 1, 1996

The doctors met with the family and told us Larry Allen may never walk or talk again.

Kim and the boys made a cassette tape to play over and over to him. The boys talked about how much they loved him and wanted him to get well, and Kim read Bible verses. They put headphones on him while he was in the coma.

December 10, 1996

We contacted family and friends to start prayer chains. There were church prayers all over the world. The doctors cut back on the medication and started to bring him out of the coma.

December 18, 1996

Once Larry A. emerged from the coma, he was moved to rehab again as an inpatient. Kim, Blaine, Jeremy, Larry Sr., and I visited daily. Larry A.'s brothers came on weekends to encourage him to walk and talk again. Larry A. started moving his arms and legs and is making sounds like he is trying to talk. He is so frustrated at losing his speech, but he knows what's going on. This is heartbreaking for all of us!

December 25, 1996

Larry Allen said "mom" on Christmas Day. That was the best gift ever. Hearing him start to talk was a miracle from the Lord.

January 24, 1997

Larry Allen came to our house to recover from the paralysis and gain strength. Kim, Ronald, and his brothers helped care for him. He started walking and talking, but the medication still causes moments of confusion. Donald took a couple of weeks of vacation to help with his care.

Larry Allen started outpatient therapy, but the doctors were unsure how successful this would be. Several months later, the doctors were amazed by his progress. Larry always worked hard to regain his skills and accepted the ones he couldn't regain.

Fridays were my day off from teaching school. I'd always take Larry Allen out for breakfast, his favorite meal, and then spend the rest of the day with him at rehab. The therapists were amazed by how hard he worked.

May 20, 1997

Eventually, Larry Allen was able to drive again. He enjoyed watching his boys play sports and taking family vacations. Larry A. and his dad took computer classes together at a local high school. Larry Allen's dream was to return to his career as a programmer/analyst; however, after taking the classes, he realized he'd lost his computer skills. He was disappointed but accepted it as God's plan. He did volunteer work at his church office.

December 26, 1997

Larry's brother Rod was getting married on a cruise ship. Most of the family on both sides flew to Orlando, Florida. We all spent the evening playing cards and having fun. On December 27, we checked into our rooms on the cruise ship, and Rod and Beth were married; Ronald was the best man, and Jeremy was a groomsman. It was a cruise to remember for a long, long time. There was a reception in one of the lounges. Larry Allen loved being with the family and had a great time.

On our return trip, we arrived at the Orlando airport only to find that all the flights to Indianapolis had been cancelled because of a snowstorm.

Since we were snowed in, we decided to make the best of it; we went sightseeing and had a great time. Those extra days of vacation were a blessing from God. He knew what we needed. Jeremy summarized it by saying, "I don't know if it was a dream or if we did all those fun things."

January 1998

Larry returned to his volunteer work at the local hospital, attended the boys' basketball games, and stayed busy with church and school.

February 1998

Several times, Larry experienced headaches and numbness in his arm; however, a steroid pill and a few days' sleep made them go away. These problems were so frustrating for him. He always questioned himself about what the triggers could be, though we all assured him he wasn't responsible—these problems were caused by the radiation he had.

The family and I always worried while waiting for the spells to pass. Would he come out of it or end up in the hospital with another big attack? It was like sitting on a time bomb. I felt so angry that he had to deal with the fear of the next attack. Hadn't he had enough loss?

March 3, 1998

Larry Allen's symptoms recurred, and he was back in the hospital, in a drug-induced coma. When he came out of the coma, they used steroids and told him to use steroid pills at the onset of a brain attack. After that, he was back in rehab, learning to walk and talk again. Larry Allen had a strong faith and never complained.

Joy comes into our lives when we have something to do, something to love, and something to hope for. He wants to help others who are sick and give them encouragement.

Struggles of the Next Five Years of Larry Allen's Life

Reoccurring brain attacks.
Dealing with tremors in his hands.
Coping with his mental and physical losses.
Paralysis.
Learning to live with his limitations.

May 2003

Larry Allen had been looking forward to summer, when the boys were out of school and he could spend more time with them. He was so proud of Blaine and Jeremy; watching them grow up was his main goal. When he had his first brain attack in August 1993, one of the things that upset him the most was the idea that he wouldn't get to raise his boys.

June 2003

I had mixed feelings when Larry Allen got in our swimming pool. I was concerned that an attack would hit while he was swimming, and we wouldn't be able to get him out. His dad and brothers kept a close eye on him, however, and we had the joy of seeing him laugh and enjoy himself. We had many pool parties and cookouts.

We had no idea that this would be our last summer with him. But we knew the attacks were coming closer together and were getting worse.

July 2003

Larry Allen, Kim, and the boys spent most of the summer on vacation. If Larry Allen started to experience any numbness or headaches, he took a steroid pill, which stopped the problem from going further. Who knew this would be the last of his vacations here on earth?

August 2003

Larry Allen finished the summer enjoying the boys, watching them get ready to go back to school. Larry Allen loved to play cards with his brothers and Larry Sr. We ended the summer by swimming and having a big cookout.

September 2, 2003

Larry Allen had a major attack and was in a coma. We talked to every doctor who'd had any success with Larry Allen's case, searching for a way to stop the attacks. The steroid pills were no longer stopping the attacks.

October 2003

Our whole family is heartbroken, seeing Larry Allen on a ventilator, being stuck with needles. *How much could his body take?* I asked myself. They brought him out of the drug-induced coma, and the seizures stopped. He was moved to a local hospital to go through rehab again. Larry Allen had an infection; the tremors were bad, and he was weak. Larry Sr. and Kim recorded Blaine and Jeremy's basketball games so Larry Allen could watch them. Kim, Blaine, and Jeremy gave him a purple pumpkin for Halloween—purple is his favorite color.

By November 2003, Larry Allen had been in the hospital for three months, and he was getting more alert. He told us he was tired of being in the hospital and of being sick. The tremors made it hard for him to feed himself, but he refused to allow any of us to feed him. He said he'd rather stop eating. He had day pass on Thanksgiving. Kim, the boys, Ron, and Hope came to our house for dinner. Larry Allen asked us if we'd found a way to stop the attacks; we told him we were still working on it. He said that if we didn't find an answer soon, he was going to die. We were heartbroken to hear him say this, but we all understood that he was worn out. I'll never forget feeling so helpless, as though we'd let him down.

December 2, 2003

Larry Allen was out of the hospital for one week. Kim took the week off, and they went to be evaluated for outpatient therapy.

December 12, 2003

Kim called and said Larry Allen was experiencing the beginning of a brain attack and that the steroids weren't working. Kim and I took Larry Allen to the hospital. He was experiencing numbness, trouble swallowing, and trouble focusing his eyes; however, he was able to talk a little, and he seemed alert when he did talk. The hospital struggled to get an I.V. started; his veins had shut down. Finally, after hours of trying, they put it in the top of his foot.

Larry A. is getting worse. He's exhausted. I asked God why he has to suffer like this.

December 14, 2003

They started the food line again. He's much more sedated. We wonder if he knows were here?

December 15, 2003

Larry's A. oxygen levels won't stay up. They want to put him back in intensive care and put a central line in his neck. They didn't allow any of us to be with him when they did this procedure. They attempted many sticks to his neck but ended up putting it in his chest. When we went in and saw his neck, we were furious—they wouldn't have been this cruel to an animal. His neck was swollen and red, and blood was gathering under the skin—then it started seeping out. We left word with our main doctor that whoever did the procedure is not allowed back in his room. To top it off, they'd sedated him, so he couldn't tell them to stop.

December 16, 2003

How many times can his body go through this? I asked myself. We set up a meeting with the primary doctors; we wanted to know their thoughts and goals. None of the doctors agreed on how to handle the case. They'd never dealt with anything like this before. Here are their thoughts and suggestions:

Put a tracheotomy in to keep the airways protected permanently.

He is no longer a candidate for rehabilitation. Put him in a long-term care facility.

His attacks will start becoming more frequent, until they are fatal.

We might want to stop all treatments and call in hospice.

We have so much to consider in this decision. Will the attacks come more frequently, until he doesn't survive? Only God knows the plans he has for Larry Allen's future. The goal is to determine what's best for Larry Allen. I remember, nineteen years ago, Larry Allen asking his dad and me not to keep him alive on machines. Our heads are spinning from all the medical options. I'm thinking about the suffering I've observed over the past nineteen years. I'll never want to give him up, but I wonder if we're being selfish at Larry Allen's expense. It feels like the bottom is falling out of my life.

December 18, 2003

Larry Sr. took pictures of Larry Allen's neck. Larry A. was responding to pain, which is a good sign. The radiation doctor came and talked to us; he said they're seeing good results from putting patients in an oxygen chamber. Larry Allen's lungs must be in good shape, so they'll test them first. The doctor said Larry A. has nothing to lose at this point. This is the first sign of any hope. We're concerned that we might not be able to get him stable enough to try this. Why weren't we told a year ago about this treatment? Could that have stopped the attacks?

December 19, 2003

I was told that Larry A.'s pneumonia is bad. They're changing the oxygen level on the vent to get him to take more breaths on his own. These are positive steps to getting him off the vent.

December 20, 2003

The nurse reported that Larry Allen's eyes followed her this morning and that, on command, he squeezed her hand. This is great; he's waking up. The pulmonary doctor came in to look over Larry A. I asked him if he was the one who'd tried to put the central line in Larry A.'s neck. He said he wasn't, but that one of his medical students was. I informed him that this was cruel to Larry A., especially since he was sedated and unable to defend himself. The doctor's reply was that Larry Allen is a hard stick. I told him that was no excuse and that he should make sure that medical student doesn't enter Larry's room again. Otherwise, we'll contact someone higher up. I don't want this to happen to another patient.

December 21, 2003

Larry A. is not responding well today.

December 22, 2003

Larry Sr. and I are so discouraged. We thought this attack was over, but Larry Allen had two seizures today.

December 24, 2003

Christmas Eve. Kim, Larry Sr., and I stayed with Larry Allen in shifts. Larry A. had several seizures today and hasn't responded to any of us. Blaine and Jeremy were able to visit, but they have a hard time seeing their dad so sick. I feel bad for the boys.

December 25, 2003

Christmas Day. Kim, Ronald, Larry Sr., and I stayed with Larry A. in shifts. Larry A. had several seizures.

December 26, 2003

Larry A. has developed a blood infection—this is bad news. His Uncle Al and Aunt Carol; his cousin Brad and Brad's wife, Koreen; and his cousin Sue came to visit. Larry Allen is not responding today, even though Brad tried hard to get him to respond. I can see how upsetting this is for all of them.

December 28, 2003

I was excited that they moved Larry A. to a room on the floor. Larry A.'s eyes are tracking when we talk to him.

January 8, 2004

I observe positive improvements daily in Larry A. He can move both arms, and Kim had a nursing home come to do an evaluation.

January 11, 2004

Larry A. had a seizure, and I wonder if another major attack is coming. Larry Allen's health over these past nineteen years has been an emotional roller-coaster ride. You get your hopes up, and then the bottom falls out again.

January 15, 2004

Kim checked on what their insurance covers for home healthcare. It will cover a nurse only for a few hours per day.

January 20, 2004

Larry A. was discharged from the hospital and taken by ambulance to a nursing home.

After work, I went to see him. His room is across the hall from the patients' smoking lounge, which isn't good on his lungs or the blood infection he already has. This is not the room they showed Kim when she checked the place out. His bed is old, and it's lying flat. Because of his pneumonia, he has to have the bed elevated. I told a nurse, but nothing was done. I assured Larry A. that we'd make new plans tomorrow. I went home and cried for leaving him there. I was worried something would happen to him. He's too sick to have sloppy care.

January 21, 2004

Larry Sr. and I went after work to check on Larry A. He was wearing the same bedclothes from the hospital, and the bed was still flat. He's alert and wants to get out of there. We asked him if he wanted to come to our house, and he said that would be great. We assured him they'd move him tomorrow. We need a hospital bed and an ambulance. His dad went home and cried at the thought of him being in the nursing home for one more night.

January 22, 2004

Kim made the arrangements to have Larry Allen moved to our house. Larry Sr. moved everything out of our office. The hospital bed and oxygen arrived, and we got everything set up. There was a mix-up with the ambulance, and it arrived around 10:00 PM. When they brought Larry A. in on the stretcher, he gave us a big smile. I hadn't seen that smile for so long. Both Larry Sr. and I knew we were in over our heads with all the shots, medicines, and food line. We were trusting that God would walk us through this process.

January 23, 2004

A home healthcare nurse came to check Larry A. over and help us. She was our angel. She taught Larry Sr. how to give the shots in Larry A.'s stomach, and we both learned tips on how to change the bed with him in it, how to manage the food line, how to manage the medicine schedule, how to roll him to prevent bedsores, and how to do the catheter. She suggested we get hospice involved, which would get us more services. She couldn't believe we'd taken this on without any training. She was supportive, though, and gave us a crash course. As Larry Allen's parents, maybe we're using our hearts to help our son and not our heads. But he's so cooperative and glad to be here.

January 25, 2004

Ron and Rod lifted Larry Allen into the wheelchair and took him into the great room. I cleaned the room and changed the bed. Kim comes after work to help with Larry A.'s care. Blaine and Jeremy come after school. Larry A. loves to see the boys and hear about their day.

February 2004

After meeting with hospice and finding out the services they provide, we switched to hospice. Larry A. was assigned a male nurse named Tom. Larry A. likes and trusts Tom; they're about the same age and have children close to the same age. They had a massage therapist come to the house, and a physical therapist worked on his muscles. They showed us how to do this daily.

Larry Sr. worked nights, while Ron and I worked days. Ron stays overnight to help with Larry A.'s care. Larry A. apologizes for not being able to take care of himself. All of us working with him tell him he'd do the same for us. We laugh and try to make anything that happens fun. Larry A. loves the fact that hospice had us stop the shots in the stomach and any more blood tests. After all these months, no one is sticking him any longer. He's able to eat certain foods by mouth, but he has to be careful not to choke. Larry Sr. reads the sports section daily with him. Kent, a friend of Larry A.'s from high school and college, came to visit and gave him the book *The Purpose Driven Life*. It's a guide to a forty-day spiritual journey. I was able to travel this spiritual journey with him. I feel blessed to have had this opportunity.

February 7, 2004

Larry Allen turned forty-two, and we had a birthday open house for friends and extended family. Family members that attended were Kim, Blaine, Jeremy, Ronald, Hope, Donald, Candise, Jason, and Brandy. Others that attended were uncles, aunts, cousins, classmates, and friends. It seems like yesterday that I had his first birthday party with friends and family. How can I let go of him? Larry Allen's high school friends made him a special birthday video.

March 2004

Larry Sr. and Ronald moved Larry Allen to his home so he could spend more time with Kim and the boys. The four of us took shifts caring for him there. He had one of his brain attacks and slept most of the time after that. He moaned in pain when he moved.

April 26, 2004

Larry Sr. spent the day with Larry A. Tom told him that the end is getting close. Larry Sr. already knew; he wondered how he'd be able to go on without him. Parents are supposed to die before their children. Larry Allen has always been a blessing in my life. I hate seeing him suffer this way, but he's going to a pain-free place: heaven.

April 27, 2004

This was my day to spend with Larry A. Kim decided she, Blaine, and Jeremy would all stay home. Tom, the hospice nurse, came and said he felt the end would come sooner than he'd thought. He told us to play Christian music, sing along with it, and hold Larry Allen's hands. When Larry A. got his wings, Kim, Blaine, Jeremy, and I played music and held his hands. Larry Sr. and Ronald arrived shortly. It is so hard to let him go, but the suffering is over. He has been fighting the disease for nineteen years. We will miss him so much—his big smile and hugs, the strong faith he had.

I know what people will say: "He's in a better place, and you wouldn't want to bring him back." But I'm screaming, "I do want him back! I want him back now!" Is that wrong? No; every parent who's lost a son or daughter knows the feeling. But we know we'll get to see Larry Allen again someday. *Our family chain is broken, and nothing seems the same; but as God calls us one by one, the chain will link again.*

Today is the tomorrow you worried about yesterday, but not nearly enough.

God saw him getting tired, and a cure was not to be.
So He put His arms around you and whispered, "Come to me."
With tearful eyes we watched you suffer and saw you fade away.
Although we loved you dearly we could not make you stay.
A golden heart stopped beating you're now at peaceful rest.
God broke our hearts to prove to us, He only takes the best.

—*Unknown*

Letter

Poem found by Larry and Delila Woodruff:

My Son

I hear your laugh; I see your smiling face. Memories…no span of time can erase.
I long to hold you close, to plant a kiss upon your cheek, but my heart can only break, my eyes can only weep.
God called you home as you reached out in one last prayer…
You now walk on "streets of gold" without an earthly care.
It would be selfish to want you back in all your pain and distress, selfish to call you away from your Heavenly happiness.
In my mind, although my heart breaks, I can always hold you close and plant a kiss upon your cheek.

****

Larry Allen became part of the Indianapolis Colts history when his family purchased a brick for the Colts Walk of Fame. It is located in the northeast plaza on Capital Avenue at "First Down" Section F.

****

Written by Hope Woodruff (Larry Allen's niece):

Uncle Larry

Uncle Larry is one of the nice guys. Always trying to help but when he was twenty-four years old he got cancer. No one knew what to do or think. That scared everyone. Now he's forty-one and has been in the hospital for fifteen weeks. He did get out for one week and went back in for two more weeks. In one week he had seven seizures.

That's bad for anyone. Sometimes the doctors will put him in a drug-induced coma for about two weeks at a time. Uncle Larry will sometimes get paralysis. That means one whole side of his body goes numb. It will even blind him in one of his eyes. Now our family takes shifts to watch over Uncle Larry at the hospital. So, everyone is trying to help. No one wants him to leave us. No one wants to leave him. We all love him very much.

The End

****

Written by Jeremy Woodruff (Father's Day 2001):

Dear Dad,

What I think is special about you is just because you are not like every other dad you don't quit being a dad. And I think that is a very important quality to life. And every time I feel down you tell me that you love me and that God is always there for me.

Here are some fond memories:

1. When you taught me how to play baseball.
2. When you taught me how to ride a bike.
3. And you let me play on the basketball team when I was too young.
4. My favorite memory is when you would act like a bull and I would try and stay on.

And I will always love you. And God will love you, too. I won't forget when you were sick and had not been awake for days and I started to rub your feet and you woke up!

So, Happy Father's Day!!!!!   Love, Jeremy!!!

Written by Jeremy Woodruff (a school report 12/10/2004):

My Hero

What makes a hero? Heroes are people who are always willing to help someone no matter what. They never give up hope, and they try to like everyone. In any situation they can stay calm and become a leader. They act first and think about the danger later. After they helped someone or whatever they don't boast about it.

The person I picked as my hero for the essay is my dad, Larry Woodruff. Now my dad wasn't exactly Superman. Don't get me wrong; I am not saying he was dumb or weak or anything like that. But he was my hero in a different way than being strong and courageous and saving me from a burning building or anything like that. But by being my dad, and a really nice, loving person, he was my hero.

Then one day in August of 1985, he was diagnosed with cancer. This was devastating to my grandparents and the whole family. But sure enough he pulled through it and was cured. But it all wasn't over. In 1996 he had his first seizure and nobody expected it. These seizures lasted for eight years until he passed away.

He and everybody else knew that he wasn't his old sports-all-star self, but we didn't care because instead of complaining about his life he was trying to make ours better. For instance when he would be sick in the hospital, he was sad that we had to come there every day and take care of him. He felt bad. My dad thought sometimes that he was a burden, but was actually very far from it.

Throughout my dad's life, he went through many challenges such as not being as strong as he use to be, going in and out of the hospital, in rehab, having cancer, and family fights.

Through all of this I never remember hearing him say "I hate this" or "my life stinks" but instead always wanting to help other people. For example, his last job was volunteering at a hospital to help other people in need. And he always loved working there especially when he got to work with kids who had cancer.

He went to Purdue to become a computer programmer, which I believe you need to be very smart to do. But when he got cancer he lost all of this and instead of getting mad he just put up with it.

So that is my hero and what I think a hero is. I think he should be the hero of the year because I know he was the hero of my life.

In loving memory of Larry Woodruff
February 7, 1962 to April 27, 2004

About the Authors

The authors Larry R. and Delila were high school sweethearts in the sixties. By the mid-seventies they had five children, including a set of twins. Larry R. worked in the computer field for thirty-five years, while Delila was a stay-at-home mom. When their last child started school, she began a thirty-year long career teaching preschool. They were very active with their boys in school, Cub Scouts, and Little League.

They lived in New Haven, Indiana, for twenty-five years and then moved to Indianapolis. They have ten grandchildren and enjoy grilling and swimming with family and friends in their backyard.

www.ingramcontent.com/pod-product-compliance
Lightning Source LLC
Chambersburg PA
CBHW020250290526

45784CB00003B/1178